the modern yoga handbook

VIJAY HASSIN

the modern Yoga handbook

A COMPLETE GUIDE TO MAKING THE SPIRITUAL AND PHYSICAL DISCIPLINES OF YOGA WORK IN YOUR LIFE

foreword by Swami Satchidananda
illustrations by Scott Cumming

Dolphin Books
Doubleday & Company, Inc.
Garden City, New York
1978

Library of Congress Cataloging in Publication Data
Hassin, Vijay.
The modern yoga handbook.
1. Yoga. I. Title
B132.Y6H327   181'.45
ISBN 0-385-13001-5
Library of Congress Catalog Card Number 77-76243

acknowledgments

There are many people who formally, and informally, have aided in the completion of this book and to whom I am deeply in debt for their contributions. First and foremost, my teacher, Sri Swami Satchidananda, for his beautiful introduction and loving support throughout this project. Secondly, my sister Jeanette Brack, for her editorial service, much of which was provided under extreme pressure. And last (but certainly not least) to my wife, Shree, for all her help. Not only did she transcribe and edit part of the manuscript, but it was she who wrote the section on Hatha yoga, women, and pregnancy. But even more important for the completion of this project, she offered continued encouragement and emotional support.

To all the seen and unseen forces who helped in the birth of this book, my eternal heartfelt thanks.

VIJAY HASSIN
NOVEMBER 26, 1977

foreword by Swami Satchidananda

Beloved Reader:

I am sure you are one of the many Yoga enthusiasts, otherwise you would not be holding a book like this one. There are many books on Yoga on the market; many talk only about certain aspects, yet very few are written to encompass all the different phases of the glorious path of Yoga. Here is one of the few.

The author is David Hassin, whom I affectionately call Vijay, meaning Victorious, because of his successful understanding of Yoga. I take pride in saying that he is one of my very loving students who has understood me and my presentations of the various aspects of this science, which I make in the name of Integral Yoga. I can easily hear myself speaking through his words throughout the book.

Yoga is not only, as many people think, a set of physical postures or the practice of silent meditation, but it is a way of life which embraces all the phases of existence. There is a yogic way of eating, sleeping, waking, drinking, a yogic way of working, learning, teaching, and relating to others. There is a yogic way of commanding and obeying, a yogic way to be a leader, and a yogic way to be a follower. This yogic way brings us to the true enjoyment and appreciation of all our experiences. Then what is this yogic way? Living a life without disturbing the peace of mind. How to obtain this peace of mind? It is not obtained, because it is our very nature. We are unable to recognize it due to a mind that is covering it by its multiple layers of disturbances. We have only to lift the layers and the peace will shine forth. This is done by eradicating from our lives all selfishness, which is the root cause of all disturbance. Yoga is a way toward selfless living which, once reached, becomes the way to live. A practitioner of this holy science is usually a peaceful, happy man.

David Hassin is in his own life a good yogi, a good student, a good teacher, a good husband, a good father, and a good friend. He is a beautiful mixture of all these, and therefore I am certain that this book by him will provide a guiding light for many seekers, that they may find their path easy and inspiring.

May the light of Yoga dispel the darkness of the world so that peace and joy may reign in the hearts of everyone.

Ever Yours in the Lord,

Swami Satchidananda

contents

CONTENTS

PART TWO — ON THE WAY IN

CONTENTS

CONTENTS

PART THREE – ON THE WAY OUT

CONTENTS

introduction

This is a book on yoga. Not just the physical postures or some "far out" psychic phenomenon but some down-to-earth basic instructions on how to start living right—right now. This is a practical book, a manual, for those who want to get started but don't know where to start. It's a book that was prompted by a lot of my students and friends over the last eleven years, running into the same problems, as well as a book of my own experiences. Many of these students had asked if there was any book to help a novice get on the Yogic Path. As there wasn't, I told them of several books that gave different aspects of the yogic or spiritual life. But many came back to say that these books didn't convey the full picture and weren't able to get them started.

That is why this book is for you, because I know how difficult it can be to want to start on a spiritual practice and not have anyone around to go to with particular questions or for advice. Hopefully, reading this book will be like having satsanga, associating yourself with spiritual people, and it can lead you out of the tight spots that often occur. There are many completely theoretical books on yoga (you can probably find them on the bookshelf right next to this one), but this isn't one of those. That doesn't mean that this book is devoid of theory; it's there, but it's mixed well in with the practices. This book is dedicated to the dictum that an ounce of practice is worth more than a ton of theory.

I have written this book in a handbooklike format which will really aid you in going to specific problems that you may have. Unlike most books, this book isn't meant to be read cover to cover but more to be browsed through. In this manner *you* will establish the plot and the direction that this book will take, as well as *your* level of understanding. There will be some things in this book you will agree with, and some you won't; some ideas in here you might even hate. All I can ask is that you keep an open mind, a mind not ready to jump and classify something one way or the other. I'm not expecting that everyone will agree with what I say; but keeping yourself open is the only way that changes can come about. And changing is what this book *is* all about. If, on the other hand, you find some things just "too weird," skip them and go on to something you can relate to. Remember, this is *your* book and *your* life.

A quick perusal of the table of contents will show you that the book is broken up into four parts: The Way, On the Way In, On the Way Out, and The Wedded Way. The first part, The Way, explains yoga and the guru in simple philosophical terms. The second, third, and fourth parts treat yoga more practically. The second part, On the Way In, is devoted to the yogic practices that lead one inward. The third part, On the Way Out, is devoted to the yogic life-style, and the fourth part, The Wedded Way, to the integration between practices and life-style. In this way, you will have a complete picture of the yogic life.

dedication

To my teacher, who showed me the path,
To my wife, who walks with me on the path,
To my parents, who prepared me for the path,
And to my friends and students, whom I meet along the path,
This book is dedicated.

part one

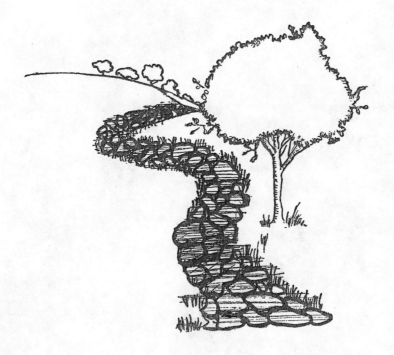

the way

chapter one — Yoga, the Vehicle

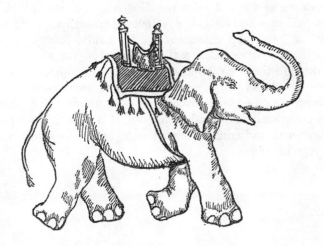

What is yoga?

It is difficult to really know what yoga is. It is quite possible that you have heard many people speak on the subject, each telling you what he individually thinks it means. And I'm sure that they sincerely wished to convey to you the *truth* about yoga. I will make no pretense of knowing what yoga is; rather, from what I have learned from my limited capacity and experience, I will simply relate to you what I think it is. At this point, let me reiterate that it is not my intent that you take everything I say as the gospel truth; rather I propose that you accept what you can and reject that which you cannot.

In talking about yoga I will often refer to God. I understand that many people may be "turned off" by that term. But God can be viewed in a variety of ways, none of them necessarily in the form or forms that society or culture has taught us to see them. Yoga is union with self, which literally means to yoke or unite the individual self with the cosmic self, God. Yogis have many meanings for God. It can be peace, infinite and all-encompassing, or it can be power; it can be bliss and joy, or even purity and all-pervading goodness. It is at the essence of God that we also find the essence of yoga. As you see, God is as difficult to define as yoga. Self can be thought of as consciousness and yoga as the means of increasing consciousness. In reality, though, you can never increase or decrease real consciousness. You are conscious, and through the yoga practices, you become more aware of that consciousness. As you become increasingly more aware, so does the awareness of consciousness grow, until ultimately you become completely and totally conscious. It is here that the process of awareness and consciousness merge, and the essence of God and yoga are one.

Yoga is a way to unite.

For many people yoga suggests physical exercises, or meditation, or possibly some exotic philosophy. It is commonly conceived of as a specific practice which is performed with regularity. Yoga is that, but much more. It is not one but a series of practices; the methods may vary, depending upon the teacher, but the goal, no matter which school of yoga you study with, remains the same: to unite the individual self with the cosmic self.

Yoga has often been referred to as a path, a way that leads you to a specific goal. However, not everybody can find the same path passable. That's why there are many paths that lead to the mountaintop so that each individual can find his own particular path, his own particular way, and consequently his own particular yoga. It is most important that each of us finds the yoga that best fits our own temperament; that is why this book was written —to give an idea of the kinds of yoga and the specific temperaments that would fit the various paths to the individual seeker.

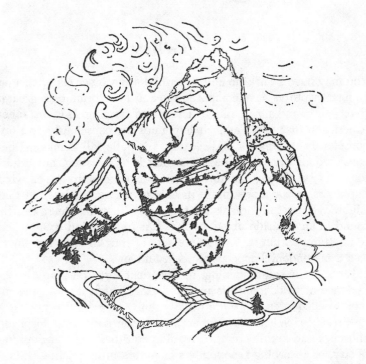

Yoga is a life of union.

Yoga, first and foremost, is a way of life. Aside from being practices and philosophy, it is a science of living. Before understanding yoga in any real sense, you must first become aware that it is life itself. Yoga is not limited to leading a proper and correct and meditative existence for short intervals of time; rather it is your whole existence. Awareness cannot be expanded for some period in the morning and rekindled again at some time in the evening; it must be expanded in all activities, in all relationships, in all capacities, and in all pursuits. That is yoga. It is nothing more than each act of the day and nothing less than life itself.

What is the Light?

You may have heard the Self described as an inner experience of Light. Scriptures have compared the Self to "a brightness greater than a thousand suns," a light that is transforming. It is this inner experience that yogis and all humanity are consciously and unconsciously striving for and seeking. I include "all humanity" because we all want happiness, one that is of a lasting, not transitory, nature. If we can throw out the old definitions of what happiness is, for more subtle meanings, we come closer to that Light. We must first disregard the notion that happiness can be found in any outside object or that it is in the mind or attached to anything within it. Rather, we should start to view happiness as a transcendental concept of peace and love.

Light is the self-sustaining, independent force that we can experience at peak moments in our lives. Though it's not uncommon to encounter it, we are usually dimly conscious or aware of its presence. When viewing artistic masterpieces and inspiring churches and architecture, or reading spiritual and transforming poetry, or absorbing the wonders of nature in its pristine beauty and awesome power, we become aware of this greatness which reaches beyond us. It is that immensity of wonder and awe encountered when we learn, through science, of the order and magnitude of the heavens, or the complexity of the human body. We feel it in the joy of seeing and holding a newborn infant whose innocence and purity are indescribable in their perfection. We know it is present in a friendship that has weathered both the joys and agonies intrinsic in sharing and giving of trust, assistance, and love. It is at such moments when we feel a force greater than ourselves that we have experienced what yogis call transfiguring Light. The Light causes a change to occur in our perceptions of the world around us. It increases our awareness, and our understanding of ourselves, by placing us in the proper relationship to truth. If you take the word understand as an example, you may see what I mean. When you try to understand, you stand under that which you are attempting to comprehend —the truth. That is what understand means; if you know that you are beneath something, you are obviously aware of its presence above you. However, many people maintain that they know the truth, that they are in essence "on top of it," standing proudly as willful conquerors. Alas, it is only through the abandonment of this stance to a more humble position that we can understand that the truth is what is above and beyond us, not below us. Only when we cease to think of ourselves as the light and life of the universe can we then abandon ourselves to that very Light and Life.

Why you can't see the Light.

The Light is difficult to see, for it is both colorless and subtle in nature. In beginning a new spiritual practice, it is often mistaken for our own particular mental attitudes and attachments. This occurs because the Light permits the shadings of these attachments and attitudes to color it. Before real spiritual practice begins, we may let our attachments to body and mind color the Light. We may feel that we are nothing more than this body, and when it departs so will we. Or we may see ourselves as a type of person, the working man, middle class, a parent, or an intellectual. These types of attachments are known as false identifications and color the Light so that it cannot be expressed purely.

In yoga we believe that these patterns of attachments are aspects of our previous lives; we must not only deal with the present but with all that has affected us—the long history of pasts, our individual karmas. (This subject will be dealt with at greater length in a subsequent chapter.)

Often circumstances occur that temporarily rip off the mask of false identity, and unprepared, we stand there dazed in the naked light. More often than not, people grope for substitutes to replace the shattered identity and keep on living the way that they have been. It is not an easy task to find your own mistakes.

Frequently, we are apt to look for the error in some circumstance or person other than ourselves. This usually helps us escape from the fact that we make the world we live in. Very often it takes only a cataclysmic event to cause us to look within and see that our attitudes have been coloring our perceptions. It is often in desperation that these changes occur; when we find that we can no longer operate in the old way, we reach out to make the first crucial step toward seeking a clearer Light, a Light without discoloration. It is at this time that active searching for a way and for a teacher who will assist in discovering a clearer Light—your own Light, the Light of a real and divine life—begins.

Aside from finding the way and the master, and clarifying your experiences so that the Light might be cleared and the discolorations removed, there is the responsibility of keeping the Light clean, a task which ultimately rests with each of us. It has often been the case that once an aspirant has been shown a clearer Light, he has failed to assume the responsibility of keeping it clean. This type of situation often results in the person experiencing a sense of guilt and oftentimes a lack of self-worth. After all, it is difficult to live with the fact that we possess the means of self-improvement, and yet find we cannot or will not use it.

chapter two — Guru, the Signpost

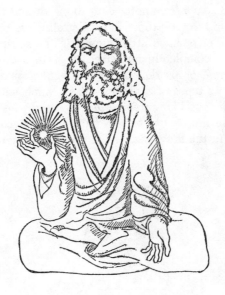

The guru, dispeller of darkness

It is said, "When the student is ready, the master will appear."
However, before we speak of a teacher, we must first decide
whether we are really ready for one. It isn't sufficient to simply
feel that you are ready for one because you think it might be
"nice" to have one—you must know definitely; then having a guru
will really mean something. Some people say gurus aren't necessary for spiritual progress; others say you won't get anywhere
without one. However, this question of whether or not to "have"
a guru is not as important as whether or not you can be a real
disciple. Gurus come and go; there are many of them; there are
few *real* disciples.

Traditionally, being a disciple of a guru was serious business. The situation appears to be quite different here in America; people put as much thought into becoming a disciple as they would into buying a pair of shoes, which are stylish today, in the closet tomorrow. It's sad, not for the guru, but for the would-be disciple; for it all stems from not seeing the guru and the guru-disciple relationship in the proper light. Certainly we do not all need a guru. Some of us have little interest in the spiritual life, while others are so completely immersed in it that they don't need gurus. The rest of us do. As Swami Venkateshananda relates, there are three types of disciples, all of which he likens to firewood. The first is like cured, dried firewood, the moment it is placed in the fire, it bursts into flames. The second is slightly damp, once in the fire it sizzles for a bit, but after drying off, it

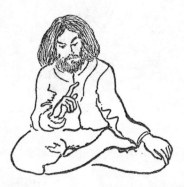

too catches. The third (with which I am quite familiar) has been left out in the rain; it is quite soaked. Even after having been placed on a raging fire, it does nothing but hiss and crackle and send up a lot of smoke. Only after considerable prodding and stoking does it finally catch. In this way, the Swami says, the three different types of disciples react to the spiritual life. Some "burst into flames" and realize God. Others need some "drying out," more effort and discipline before they "catch." And still others need a great deal of "prodding," sometimes a lifetime of unstinting devotion to the practices, before they finally "catch."

Gurus are not necessary for the first type, sometimes not even for the second, but for the third, they are indispensable. Gurus provide a constant source of energy and, if used properly, they will show you how to "light *your* fire." "Gurus are signposts," my teacher has often said; they will point out the way, but we have to walk the distance.

I realize that you may not want a guru; you may consider him the farthest thing from your life. But an honest discussion of the guru and the guru-disciple relationship is necessary; for if you do all or any of the things that will be described in the following chapters, they will inevitably lead you to a guru, a signpost.

The guru's many forms.

The guru, the dispeller of darkness, can take the appearance of one of many different forms. It may be an enlightened personality in a living, physical form; it may be a physical personage that has passed away (Christ, Buddha, a great saint or sage). It may be some scriptures (Koran, Bible, Bhagavad Gita), or it may even be the man next door. When we talk of gurus, we are usually referring to signposts that direct us within. However, when we speak of the real Guru, we are referring to that Light which all these smaller gurus reflect. The practices and the teachings of any spiritual discipline will make us aware of the many gurus around us, and thus we will be able to take fuller advantage of their presence. They will be like allies, ready to aid in our search within. That search ultimately ends at the feet of the real Guru.

Now you are at the beginning of your journey; maybe you are not even aware that you are on a journey. Well, you are. Just picking up this book and glancing at it indicates some interest in the spiritual life. The cultivation of that interest is for now your guru, your signpost leading you in. You can view your interest in yoga that way, or you can study it as an exercise in intellectual curiosity, one signpost among many. The key to understanding the guru is to realize that it looks like anything or anyone else, but the truth is only seen from the eyes of the seeker. For the guru is a mirror, showing you exactly what you project on it. If you project a man or a woman, that's what he will show you; if you project fear or anger, that's what you will see. How many people read Lord Jesus's message in the Bible, each arriving at a different interpretation? How many sects and approaches are there in Buddhism?

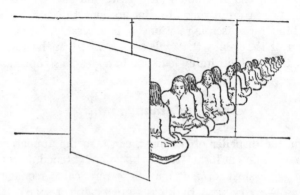

As a guru is a perfect mirror, so it enables you to see your imperfections. Only when you are free from these imperfections can you really see the guru. If you placed two mirrors face to face, and stood in the center between them, you would be able to see your reflection bounce off the two of them into infinity. Such is the case with two who know one another, for in reflecting each other's perfect clarity, they are echoing infinitely.

At the start of our journey it is helpful to have some guidance, though it isn't absolutely necessary. However, if you feel you don't need the help of a guru, or that this guru business is silly, disregard the rest of the chapter and go on to the next. Remember, this is your book; use it to your capacity.

Will the true guru please stand up?

Some people, in their enthusiasm in finding their guru, launch on a propaganda campaign for their teacher, a quite natural occurrence among beginning aspirants. They feel that they have found not only the true teacher, but the true way, and in their excitement, they want to share it with everyone they know. They will implore you to see their teacher and try their particular way, unceasingly bombarding you with long quotations from their teacher. It is not odd to find that in speaking about the teachings, they will constantly interject what their guru has said about "this and that." Some, in their zeal, will go as far as stating that their guru is the "true teacher," the conveyor of "true yoga." Finally, they may even recite some spiritual or mystical "mumbo jumbo," claiming in the same breath that there can be only a certain number of true teachers on the earth at one time and that they have found one. If, in reality, you were searching for a teacher, you might, in all probability, hear various disciples of different teachers each saying exactly the same thing about their guru. This can be both confusing and tiresome but understandable if seen in the proper light. Any teacher that you choose for yourself is your true guru. There may be a teacher who has many students, all finding him to be their true guru; however, that does not mean that everyone should follow and study under this particular master. If that were so, there would exist only one or two gurus, but there are many, and they come in all sizes and shapes, with variant approaches that appeal to different people. When the student finds a guru that fits him, he is often lead to the erroneous belief that his "perfect fit" is also suitable for everyone else. In practice it has been seen that even the greatest teachers do not suit all of us. In searching for the true guru, you are really looking for yourself. And in order to find yourself, you must first find a mirror of your perfect self, and that will become your teacher. Thus the search for the true guru must be an individual venture.

The necessity for a guru, or, I need help.

When you can no longer handle the spiritual practice on your own, and you find the need for personal guidance, you have reached the point that the famous adage alludes to, "When the student is ready, the master will appear." It cannot be emphasized enough that the call for help must be genuine and the feeling of the aspirant be not one of a dilettante, but rather of a sincere seeker. Often we've seen cartoons depicting an aspirant in search of a guru sequestered in a cave high in the Himalayas. Certainly, most of us do not have to go to the high reaches of the Himalayas to find a teacher. But your attitude and sincerity should reflect the premise that you would do that if it was necessary. You must be both sincere and willing to change your life in order to come under the tutelage of a teacher.

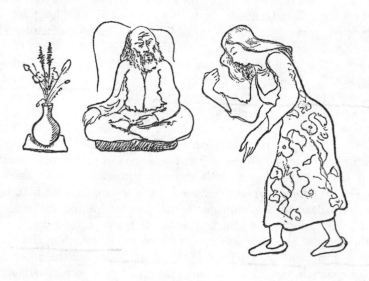

Relationship between the guru and disciple.

In order to understand the relationship between the guru and the disciple, we must first know the various levels of teacher-student associations. Disciple, aspirant, seeker, and devotee are all terms to denote the various levels of intensity of a spiritual student. Whereas the disciple is one who is already on the path of yoga, the aspirant is one who is just beginning to get established on that path, still closely following the instructions of a teacher. Seekers are those disciples or aspirants actively questing for the Truth, and devotees are those disciples or aspirants more or less emotionally bound to a particular spiritual path and/or teacher. Disciples and aspirants may start off and remain devotees, but not all will evolve quickly to become seekers. Often you see devoted aspirants making the mistake of treating and acting toward teachers as equals. This is a clear sign that they are not yet ready for a full relationship with the teacher, for one of the prime attitudes that a disciple has toward his master is humility. However, in America, where we are raised with the theoretical ideal that we are all equal, we find it repugnant to place anyone above ourselves. Thus it is shocking to many to see disciples, particularly American disciples, bowing their head to the feet of a guru, who many may see as merely another person. But, as you will see, the disciple does not view the guru in this manner. As the true disciple develops, he sees the guru less as a person and more as the true spirit personified. He realizes that if he is to understand, he must stand under the guru, he must humble himself. In this way, he tries not to block the guru's spirit by his own coloration nor his own ego attachments. The disciple tries to remain a receptive vehicle for the guru's teaching. He realizes that unless he empties himself, he cannot receive that teaching. There is a wonderful Zen story of a proud young aspirant who went to a master for the first time. Upon seeing the student, the master, without saying a word, invited him for some tea. The lad happily started chatting about his accomplishments to the master, and as they were talking the teacher dutifully poured the lad a cup of tea. But instead of filling it and stopping, the master kept on pouring. The student stared in amazement as the tea brimmed over the top. Finally unable to contain himself, he blurted out, "Master, it's filled to the top; you can't put in any more." The teacher stopped and looked up, "And so it is with you, my son. You are filled to the brim with your own ideas and self-importance. I cannot give you anything until you empty yourself first." Especially for American aspirants, the greatest

[margin annotation: So filled with self importance.]

ego attachment to <u>overcome is pride</u>. Imagine the difficulty of a first meeting between a well-educated, moderately wealthy American and a half-clad, penniless Indian, whose looks and actions are strange and foreign to the aspirant. Carlos Castañeda had very much the same experience with his teacher, Don Juan.

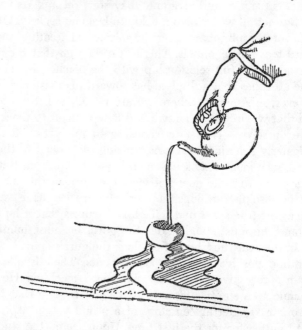

It took many years before Carlos realized that his pride was detouring him from fully understanding not only what Don Juan was teaching but, more importantly, what he was saying. <u>Cutting through pride and self-importance is a major step</u> in the relationship between guru and disciple. Early in their association, the guru will impart many ideas and precepts to his student, but only after many hearings and subsequent meetings does the aspirant begin to sniff at the scent of Truth. Oftentimes, the guru relates many different thoughts, but beneath all these ideas remains the constant, what he is really saying. And what he is saying is not translatable into words; rather, it is an inner message, an inner communication that is perceived when the defenses, blocks, and attitudes are down, or diminished. This is why the disciple humbles himself before the guru; for he will never hear what the guru is saying unless he is able to do that.

Guru worship.

We will briefly discuss this subject here and, later on, cover it more extensively in the Bhakti yoga section. In many yogic paths, disciples use the guru as an object of worship, as a deity. There are many practices disciples perform in worshiping their guru. These practices are frequently misinterpreted as acts of investing the power of God in a man. Certainly, there are some disciples who only worship the body, "the person," of the guru; however, the true intent of the practice is the student's devotion to the guru's indwelling spirit. It is that spirit that the true disciple perceives in his worship of the guru. There are some formal rituals that can be done to the guru, like using the guru as the main deity in a puja—ritual worship. (See Heart Work.) But the major intent of these formal worships should never be to focus on the body or personality, but on the indwelling spirit. In short, guru worship is just that, supplication to the guru's spiritual essence.

Guru service.

Guru service is an important aspect of the disciple's practice. Just as guru worship is a part of Bhakti yoga, the devotional aspect of yoga, guru service is one part of Karma yoga, the selfless action aspect of the yoga practice. The disciple tries to become a perfect channel; or, as many teachers phrase it, an instrument for the Lord's (or the cosmic power's) work. To be that instrument, to evolve so that you can feel the supreme power working through you, you must first become selfless and purely motivated; then you will become free to do what the Lord dictates. This is far from being an easy task; often aspirants misconstrue what they are doing as God's work, when in essence they are serving themselves. Here lies one of the significant roles of the guru; he clarifies the disciple's thinking process. A frequent method he uses is to give the disciple, if he so wants it, work to do. He then watches the disciple perform his tasks. Some will take their jobs seriously and perform them meticulously, others will take their jobs lightly and perform them sloppily, while still others will simply forget about them altogether. The guru watches and closely observes this activity and then, at the proper moment, reminds the disciples of what they are doing. Usually at this time, the aspirant is brought to the realization that, in fact, he has been led by his own mind, his own viewpoint, his own bad habits, and, alas, his own inclinations. If the aspirant is properly oriented, he will soon be wondering whether he will ever be capable of executing the demanding work of God, if he is finding difficulty performing the *simple* tasks of the teacher. He is, however, making one error in judgment, that of considering the tasks of the guru simple; for in yoga, what may suggest simplicity on the surface is usually far more exacting and complex underneath. This reminds me of the story of Milarepa, the great Tibetan yogi, who was asked to build a house for his teacher Marpa. The teacher told him the specifications of how he wanted it built. After the arduous and long task was completed, the teacher came back, looked at the house, told Milarepa that it was done all wrong and that he must start from scratch again. Milarepa proceeded to do as he was told; he tore the house down and built another. The teacher came back a second time and again told him that it was still wrong and should be torn down. Down again it went and up went another one. This situation repeated itself several times over a period of many years, until Milarepa, with sores covering his hands and body and completely exhausted, finally achieved what the teacher wanted. At which point Milarepa asked the teacher, "Why did you make me go through all this?" The teacher's explanation was simple and exact, "The point was not to build the house but that you learn

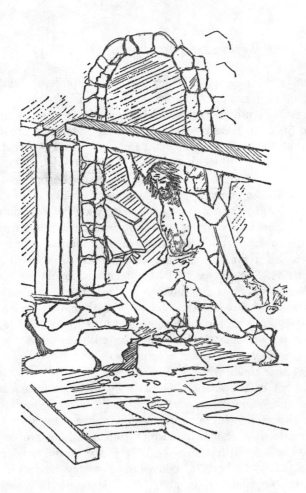

of humility and humbleness through menial work." Few people have to go to such extremes to learn humility; however, Milarepa was an extraordinary yogi, and his teacher had to give him extraordinary practices to reveal his disciple's brilliant nature. Although we are unlikely to receive such austere practices today, certainly what the guru does request of us is often just as vexing.

Trying to figure the guru out.

Aspirants and disciples alike expend considerable amounts of time trying to figure out the guru and/or what he's "up to." It is an interesting study, one which I have frequently found myself engaged in. I can honestly say that, although you may *think* you know what the guru is doing, you invariably find out that you don't. My teacher often quotes the Tamil expression, "Only the snake knows the feet of a snake," to illustrate the problem and the answer to the guessing game. As only one snake truly knows all the mechanisms of another snake, so only a guru will know the ways and means of another guru. One moment the guru will seem to be a sane, rational, and reasonable man; the next he'll appear to be a crazy, irrational, and totally incomprehensible human being. Sometimes, he'll be a pleasant, lovely individual; other times, he'll be comparable to a raging tiger. One day you will do something which he will extol with public praise; the next day you may do the same thing, but instead you will receive a torrent of condemnation, leaving you with an acute sense of shame. Gurus vary in severity; some beat their disciples, others verbally abuse them, while still others will go as far as throwing disciples out of the ashram. Gurus vary in their accumulation and use of money; some have huge bank accounts and spend lavishly; others are without a cent and are always begging. Some are as modern as the most current trends, others are as old-fashioned as a worn tradition, and there is even a third kind of guru, he that looks both to today and yesterday for inspiration. They are stingy and rich, loving and scornful, like magnets whose poles are constantly being changed in reference to the disciple, sometimes attracting, other times rejecting. These are the gurus to look for, because they will drive a disciple to distraction and ultimately to bliss. There is no means or method to figure out these gurus because they encompass the dualities and use them as tools to drive the disciples out of their own traps of dualistic distinctions.

Letting the guru work on you.

It is not simply enough to present yourself to the guru; in order for the guru-disciple relationship to come to fruition, you must surrender to him. Some find this an easy process; others discover it to be quite difficult. Nevertheless, if the guru is to do any real work with, and on, the disciple, the disciple must give himself wholeheartedly. What this means varies with both the student and the teacher. There are spiritual organizations where the students are extremely deferential to the teacher. They may do this through subtle attitudes or ritualized behavior. In India, it is not uncommon for the student, upon meeting the teacher, to kneel down and put his head at the guru's feet. Many Westerners think this form of genuflection is not only desired by the teacher, but enforced by him. This is not at all the case; the student is the one who is anxious to perform this action of humility. In this way he is expressing his desire to surrender himself up to the teacher. There are other esoteric meanings for putting one's head to the teacher's feet. The most commonly known is the belief that human beings are like large bar magnets, with the head being thought of as the North Pole, and the feet the South. The student, anxious for some of the power that the teacher possesses, attracts it by putting his North Pole (head) to the teacher's South Pole (feet). Yogis believe that the head, the hands, and the feet are great receivers of energy. (See pranayama in Body Work and Mind Work.) The hands and the feet are also good direct transmitters of energy.

As a rule, humility and obedience are the hallmarks of a good disciple. No real teacher will expect these submissions to be immediately forthcoming. Most students are skeptical when they first encounter a teacher; they wish to find out whether he is a *real* teacher and whether his ways of teaching are good and proper ones. A teacher will see this and respect it. A student eventually reaches a point in his development when he must decide whether the teacher and his methods are proper for him. He cannot continue and be a naysayer forever; he must, after all, make a decision. Once that decision has been made, the student should adapt to the guru and, in all humility and obedience, attempt to follow his teachings. And for his part, the teacher will work very carefully and meticulously on the student through his instructions.

Guru as model.

There is a story about the great teacher Shankaracharya, who, on a hot day, was walking down a dusty road, with his disciples following close behind. He was extremely thirsty and asked all the disciples, "Where can I find something to drink? I'm so thirsty, I don't care what it is." They, however, could find nothing for him. After walking for a short distance he encountered a man going in the opposite direction. He said to the man, "Do you have anything to drink?" "No, nothing but some liquor," the traveler responded. "Okay, I don't care, just give it to me; I'm much too thirsty to quibble," he said as he partook of some of the alcoholic beverage, to the astonishment of all. The disciples, upon seeing the guru do this, asked the man for some also. Shankaracharya silently looked back and watched what the disciples were doing. After they had all taken a drink, they resumed their walk and soon reached a town at the edge of the road. Shankaracharya immediately went to the blacksmith's shop. There was a crucible of molten iron resting at the edge of the blazing furnace. The guru walked up to the blacksmith and made the same request that he had made to the man on the road. However, before the blacksmith could give Shankaracharya some water, he picked up the burning crucible of liquefied iron and swallowed some of the contents. Everyone watched in dumbfounded amazement. He then turned to the disciples and offered them some. "You wanted a drink; drink this." They all responded in a rush, "We can't swallow that; it would burn us to bits." "Ah," said Shankaracharya, "but before when I had some liquor, you decided you could do that. Disciples cannot do what the master can do. Even if it looks as if you can, you can't." This may be somewhat of a strange story with which to begin this section, but I particularly wanted to illustrate how careful you must be in picking up on aspects of the guru that you wish to use as models. Certainly, on some days, the guru will act so unpredictably that it seems im-

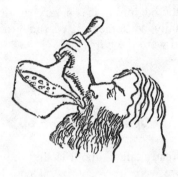

possible to follow anything he does. However, on the whole, there are aspects of his personality and entire being that you should emulate. For first and foremost, the guru is a perfected being, and it is this ideal aspect that you should look toward, follow, and have standing at the core of your conceptual knowledge of him. It is the disciple's task to pierce through the guru's body and personality and find out what makes him a perfect living being. When you have discovered and struck that essence in him, you will know that you are closely coming upon that which you should emulate and follow. Frequently, novice students will copy the teacher's speech mannerisms and dress in the style of clothes that he wears. They will walk in a gait similar to his and recite to others the same stories that he has told them. In other words, they will become like the guru, but only in body and personality. This, in a way, is an attempt by the students to use the teacher as a model, but what they are modeling themselves after is not really the teacher; it is only his accouterments, his outermost shell. In the beginning, this is not bad, and it is understandable. It is an attempt by the beginning student to internalize the guru. Since the student is still somewhat gross in his perception, all he will see to emulate will be those grosser aspects of the guru. But after some time, the student will not need to hold on to these aspects because he will have struck a level of commonality between the guru and himself that will be real and unchanging. This level of commonality is what draws the student to the guru. In the beginning it is a very subtle flame, but as one evolves, it virtually consumes all of the grosser characteristics that one believed were the guru.

Opening yourself up.

Now we have already talked about letting the guru work on you. And I guess if we were to categorize, it could be put under the heading of self-surrender, because when you surrender, you are allowing yourself to be worked on by the guru, or the divine forces around you. But what happens when you don't have a guru? You have to open yourself up to those cosmic forces which can be your teacher until one actually arrives. I remember hearing a teacher say that it is hard for an eighty-year-old who has never smiled to learn that simple act of showing pleasure. It is far easier, he reasoned, for a young person to learn to smile, because he has so much less to overcome. Opening up, letting go, and allowing yourself to flow are all ways that you can increase your sensitivity to things that are happening within and around you. It is an absolute necessity for a beginning student to develop this sensitivity. If the student does not have it, teacher upon teacher can pass before him, and he will never be able to recognize them as such. That is what is meant by the saying, "When the student is ready, the master will appear." Unless the student has worked on himself first, and has achieved a certain degree of perception, he could not and would not be ready for a teacher, even if he was standing directly in front of him.

Introspection.

Introspection, or self-analysis, is an additional aspect that the beginning student should cultivate, in preparation not only for the teacher, but also for any future spiritual study. Analyzing your motives and actions are very important steps in learning about yourself. It helps you understand what you are doing and develops an indwelling, or indrawn, attitude; it starts the process of detaching the mind from objects of the world and placing it more securely on the self. Take, for instance, the teacher-aspirant situation. If an aspirant is constantly running after worldly objects, he will find that he is disrupting his ability to see or understand what the teacher is saying. He will tend to look beyond the teacher, thinking that the truth lies somewhere outside his sphere. He will analyze the teacher from the references of his own worldly experiences, seeing him as another object and judging him accordingly. And this is a great and ignominious mistake, because a teacher cannot be judged by standards of this world. In any case, the aspirant's attention is misdirected; he should not be judging anyone, no less the teacher, but rather analyzing himself to find out about those particular aspects of his life that keep causing him distress and pain. And further, he should be asking himself the extremely important question, "Why do I do things that give me pain?" It is this type of self-analytical questioning, along with the removal of the pain-producing obstacles, that helps give the aspirant a clearer view of himself and the world. The third criteria that comes into play now is the aspirant's admission to himself that he truly desires to make the spiritual plunge and look within. Here is an example of how this deep-felt, gut desire takes hold. Always at some stage in the development of the aspirant, the tremendous personal psychic pain becomes unbearable. The student cries out for help; he has tried everything, and nothing has worked. He may have tasted of the world's pleasures, yet none have given him enjoyment. Perhaps he has had money, power, luxury, intellect, but none of these were able to quell the battle that is going on within him. It is at this point, when the aspirant finds that whatever he leans on crumbles beneath his weight, that he turns in on himself to find some long-awaited and lasting inner peace. This does not happen to all aspirants. There are some that turn within naturally; however, it has been my experience that most students have made the decision to look inside themselves after they have exhausted all the outside possibilities.

Dedicating yourself to the task.

Once one has decided to turn within, dedication to the task usually follows. It is that first little taste of peace that you experience which becomes the impetus for further spiritual efforts. And this requires as sincere a dedication as anything else in the spiritual or, for that matter, temporal realms. We have all heard about the great achievements brought about by people of great determination and dedication. They are represented in so many fields of interest: science, exploration, the arts, journalism, sports. And I must reiterate, as dedication is a necessary ingredient in the aforementioned spheres, so it is in the spiritual life. Without it, nothing can be achieved. A guru looks for people with dedication. He does not expect them to come to him as completely devoted people; however, they should exhibit some aspect of a spiritual pledge. Often, an individual who is dedicated in another endeavor, will be a dedicated spiritual student as well. So the four things necessary for a student in preparing either for a guru, or God, are self-surrender, introspection, sincere desire, and dedication. Nothing can be achieved without these four very important attitudes.

part two

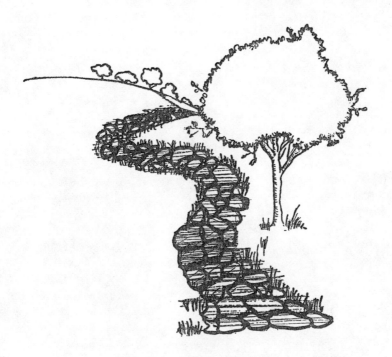

on the
way in

chapter one — Body Work, A Clean Machine

Preventive maintenance.

Now I believe it is appropriate for us to turn to the practices of Hatha yoga, the physical school of the yoga system. At the onset, before we get into the theory and practice of Hatha yoga, it would be beneficial for us to look at some of the often neglected aspects of physically working with our bodies. There is a large growing awareness of physical culture and sports participation in the American contemporary scene. People are pursuing physical activities to improve the tone of their bodies, or build up their sagging muscles, and to feel and look better and healthier. These are worthwhile activities that should be part of everyone's daily regimen. In today's society, where so much is done for us by machines, we find that we perform little if any strenuous exercise. Technology has separated us from those "bygone years" when people had to work long, hard days in the fields, growing the food they needed for subsistence. Then, there was no thought to exercise; existence provided all that was necessary. Therefore, for today's bodies to run as efficiently as yesteryear's, extra things, exercises, must be performed. Like cars, they must be run regularly to burn out and rid themselves of the sludge deposits that build up. If a car stands idle too long, or is merely taken out for short trips to the supermarket, it tends to accumulate carbon deposits in its cylinders. This causes knocking in the engine and backfiring; in other words, the machine is performing less than perfectly. Mechanics recommend for this malady a long run to burn out these harmful deposits. So the same care and treatment should be given to your body. As a machine, it too must be taken care of, looked after, and even cleaned of its sludge. It should be neither overworked nor underrun. It should be fed the proper fuel in sufficient quantities. It should be kept in tune as you, the user of your body, would be attuned to its needs and condition, looking and listening for the slightest rattles or rumbles, making sure it is in proper functioning order. Essentially, you would be practicing what mechanics call "preventive maintenance," making certain that little problems don't balloon into big troubles. Many people are taking care of their own automobiles with the aid of automotive manuals which provide step-by-step instructions for handling most mechanical difficulties. Hatha yoga, too, is a program of preventive maintenance. It leads you into an overall awareness of your body, a how-to method of treating it properly; eat the proper foods but don't overeat; exercise but don't forget about relaxing. Hatha yoga is designed to let you become aware of the body and to test out those things that make it feel good and healthy. Hatha yoga can benefit anyone, any age, and any physical type. One does not need to be healthy to practice Hatha yoga; however, one does need a healthful attitude that is receptive to the potential that it brings to the practitioner.

Proper attitude.

Attitude, though you might not expect it, is an integral and significant part of the practice of Hatha yoga. Many people, not only in Hatha yoga practice, but in other physical culture practices, go into the various postures or perform specified exercises because they are unhappy with their bodies; they neither like the way they look nor how they feel. Frequently, this is a very good motivating force; however, there are often underlying causes, feelings that encompass more than the physical appearance of the body. To put it precisely, people often dislike their bodies because they dislike themselves, and they project this image onto their bodies. This being the case, no physical culture (Hatha yoga included) can give them the bodies they seek. If perfection rests only in the mind, it doesn't matter how flawless the body is; it will always be seen as imperfect. Another problem is that people often compare and judge their bodies against the standard presented by the American commercial image. Television, news-

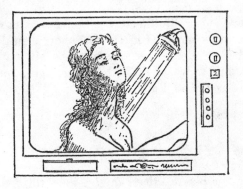

papers, and magazines broadcast this image as the model all Americans should emulate. Not everybody's physical type can or should fit this commercially packaged image. And why should we even strive for such a "goal"? We pride ourselves on individuality in thought; why not also in appearance? This reminds me of a program I saw a while back extolling the virtues of the obese individual. Perhaps that might be slightly overblown, but it is certainly the case in our society today that the overweight or even plump person is viewed as an anomaly. I'm sure heavy people are subtly discriminated against in social circumstances. The underlying message of our culture and the media that translates it is that happiness lies in possessing a "perfect" body. Our movie stars, and even some of our politicians, are admired for the "perfectness" of their physical forms. In order to practice Hatha yoga, you must rid yourself of this terribly constricting model of what a body should look like. Rather, you should accept your body type, whether it be fat, thin, or in-between, and proceed at that point to do the practices. Let the practices help you decide what kind of body is naturally and comfortably yours. It shouldn't matter what your body looks like if your health is good and your mind is at peace. We are seeking our own natural states, and there are no preconceived models in our search, merely guidelines to help us find our own internal models. You will find that your model will constantly be in a state of change and modification, until ultimately it becomes as useless and unnecessary as a woolen coat in Death Valley; then, like the coat, you will shed it. Remember, Hatha yoga will not give you a model of a slim, trim body; it will, however, give you a model of a healthy, relaxed, and flexible body.

A little theory.

Hatha yoga is a practice that can give the individual real health by toning up the musculature and the endocrine and nervous systems. It also prepares the body for long periods of meditation by making the anatomy flexible and strong enough to sit in one pose for a considerable length of time. The postures calm the mind by relaxing the body. This is done through regular, rhythmic breathing. I reiterate, Hatha yoga is a diagnostic tool. Through the practices of Hatha yoga, you become increasingly more aware of your body; with this acquired awareness, you can practice preventive maintenance, keeping the body tuned by proper diet and regular physical exercise.

The nervous systems.

Yogis believe there are two nervous systems, the gross one which we all know of and the more subtle one, called nadis, which operate in the astral body. These nadis collect into seven centers along the physical spine. The most important nadis are the Ida (pronounced Eeda), the Pingala, and the Sushumna, which operate along the whole length of the spinal cord. These three nadis intertwine at the seven centers, or chakras. These chakras are located more or less on the physical body at the base of the spine; just below the genitals; at the navel; at the heart; at the base of the throat; between the eyebrows; and at the top of the head. The Sushumna only functions when the divine subtle force, called the kundalini or the serpent power, rises through the different chakras, giving the practitioner more intense visions until it reaches the highest chakra, whereupon the individual achieves samadhi, or bliss-consciousness.

Through the postures and the breathing exercises, both the gross and the subtle nervous systems are calmed, toned, and strengthened. Good appetite, sleep, mental attitude, are in the hands of the Hatha yogi. Postures prepare you for deeper, more powerful experiences in meditation by strengthening the nerves and getting them ready for an increase in energy. Hatha yoga itself should not "kick off" a kundalini experience; kundalini raises naturally when the student has purified himself not only physically, but mentally as well.

The endocrine system.

The yoga practices not only tone up these very important glands, but help regulate them through the control of prana, or life force. When the Hatha yogi learns to control prana, he or she can control their thoughts and movements and, by doing that, indirectly control the functioning of these glands. Several poses like the shoulder stand and fish pose use glands as focal points of concentration.

Some hints.

Age No restrictions, but no matter what age, there should be no straining. Beginners should take it slow and easy.

Women Generally it is advised to discontinue yoga practice during the menstrual period, because of the discomfort it may cause. Some advanced practitioners find this to be a bit cautious. All I can say is not having a woman's body, I would not know; try for yourself and see. Later on there is a separate section on exercises for pregnancy.

Children The advanced poses should not be encouraged. Stick to the simple ones and make it loose and enjoyable. Children have great imaginations; use it in conjunction with the poses.

The bowels When beginning yoga practice, it is good to have the bowels evacuated. Those starting for the first time can take an enema; this helps purify the system. Those who have a difficult time evacuating the bowels in the morning can take a cup of warm water and gently massage the abdomen.

Time Best in the morning, but prepare to be stiff; everyone is. If you get discouraged easily, or don't have the time, you can do it in the afternoon; you will be looser then. When you do yoga postures in the morning, you feel the effects throughout your day.

Place and dress Have a blanket or a mat to do your poses on. It should be soft, but not mushy. You can put a towel over it. Find a place where you will be free from distractions and will have plenty of air and light. Your dress can be simple and light—leotards and tights for women; shorts or loose pajamalike pants for men.

BODY WORK, A CLEAN MACHINE

Breathing Remember to breathe! Keep it through the nose, unless otherwise instructed, and let it flow naturally. Some poses will constrict the breathing; take small breaths at that point.

Eating Don't eat for at least two hours before practicing the postures, nor for one half hour after.

Physical exercises These can be done in conjunction with a Hatha yoga program, but never mix up the two. Try to separate them by doing the Hatha in the morning and the exercises in the evening. If that can't be done, then do the exercises first, then wait for a while and do the postures last.

One-upmanship Never do the poses as a stunt or to show how good you are. This is a real perversion of an ancient and esoteric science.

The class.

Since this is a practical rather than theoretical book, I have provided a sample Hatha yoga class; most descriptions of postures are accompanied by illustrative diagrams. If you have a tape recorder, you can record this sample class, thus providing yourself with a regular Hatha yoga class whenever you want. The diagrams illustrate the poses, as well as specify the areas of the body and the organs that are massaged and stretched. Benefits, too, are listed. This sample class exemplifies my own particular philosophy about Hatha yoga; experience is more significant than theory.

sample hatha
yoga class

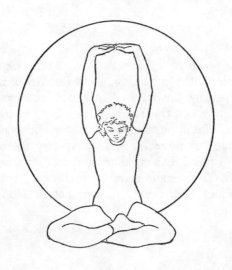

Close your eyes.
Have a straight back.
Breathe naturally. (Wait 10 seconds.)
Inhale and chant *OM* three times.

Eye exercises
nethra vyayamam

Keep your eyes closed unless otherwise instructed.
The first thing we'll be doing is eye exercises.
Straighten your back again.
Now we'll be taking the eyes straight up and straight down.
Open the eyes.

Up, down.
Up, down.
Up, down.
Up, down.   (12 seconds.)
Up, down.
Up, down.
Close the eyes.   (Rest 10 seconds.)

Next we will take the eyes from the right to the left.
Keep the head still.
Open the eyes.

Right, left.
Right, left.
Right, left.
Right, left.   (12 seconds.)
Right, left.
Right, left.
Close the eyes.   (Rest 10 seconds.)

Now on the diagonal, from the upper right corner to
the lower left corner.
Open the eyes.

Upper right, lower left.
Upper right, lower left.
Upper right, lower left.
Upper right, lower left.　　　　　　　(12 seconds.)
Upper right, lower left.
Upper right, lower left.
Close the eyes.　(Rest 10 seconds.)

Okay, now on the opposite diagonal.
Open the eyes.

Upper left, lower right.
Upper left, lower right.
Upper left, lower right.
Upper left, lower right.　　　　　　　(12 seconds.)
Upper left, lower right.
Upper left, lower right.
Close the eyes.　(Rest 10 seconds.)

Also remember to keep the mouth closed.

Now we'll be doing a full clockwise circle, touching all
4 points of the eye socket, keeping the head still.
Open the eyes.

Start at the upper right corner.
Come down to the lower right,
Across to the lower left,　　　　　(15 seconds.)
Up to the upper left,
And across to the upper right.

Now take it at your own rate, touching all four points.
Try to roll the eye around, touching the furthest periph-
ery of the eye socket that it can.
Stretch it out, down, and up.
Keep the head still, just move the eyes.
Close the eyes.　(Rest 10 seconds.)

Now we'll take the eyes in the opposite direction, counterclockwise.
Open the eyes, starting at the upper-left corner.
Go around counterclockwise.
Keep the head still.
Really stretch the eyes out.
Close the eyes. (Rest 10 seconds.)

Keep the eyes closed.
Rub the palms together, building up some heat in the palms. Rub them briskly.
Now cup the palms over the eyes, finger tips touching the hairline.
Keep the eyes closed, and feel the energy which you created by rubbing the palms together, pranic energy coming off the palms, and relaxing and rejuvenating the eyes.
Keeping the eyes closed, bring the palms down over the face, finger tips lightly gliding over the face, out toward the ears.
Gentle strokes, really soft, just as if you were washing away all the tiredness in the eyes.
Now bring the palms down over the face, into the lap.
Straighten up the spine.
Breathe naturally.

Total time: 3.8 minutes. As you become more proficient, increase the length of time on each eye exercise.)

Sun worship
soorya namaskaram

Now open your eyes and stand up.
We'll be doing Sun Worship, Soorya Namaskaram.
Sun Worship is a series of twelve poses done as one:

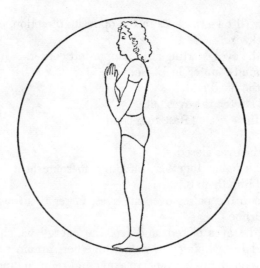

The palms come together.   (3 seconds.)

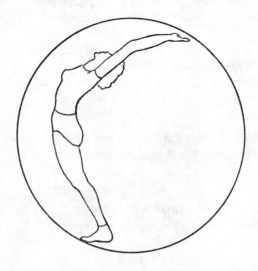

Hook the thumbs behind, over the head, and stretch
back. Look back.   (8 seconds.)

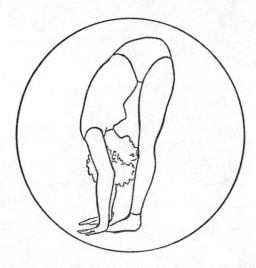

Palms come to either side of the feet, head to the knees. (8 seconds.)

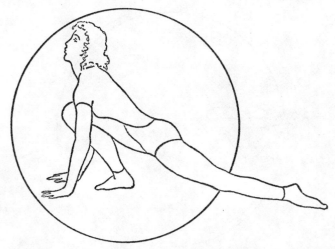

Left leg back, left knee down on the floor, head up. Right foot should be in between the palms. (15 seconds.)

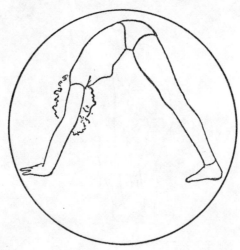

Both feet back, buttocks are raised up as the apex of a triangle. Heels are stretching to the floor. (15 seconds.)

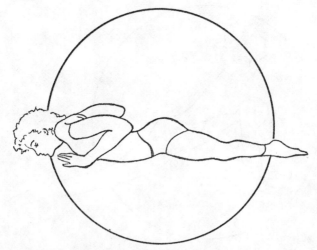

Knees, chest, and chin. Knees come to the floor, chest comes to the floor, and chin comes to the floor. Feet are flat on the floor. The buttocks are slightly raised. (15 seconds.)

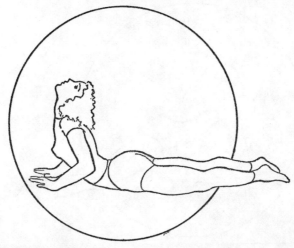

The pelvis comes down; the head, neck, and shoulders come up. (7 seconds.)

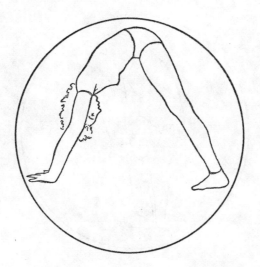

Come back to the heels, triangle position. (7 seconds.)

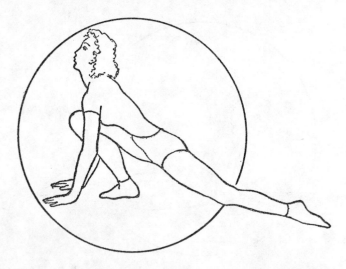

Left foot in between the palms in one step. Right knee down on the floor, and the head up.   (15 seconds.)

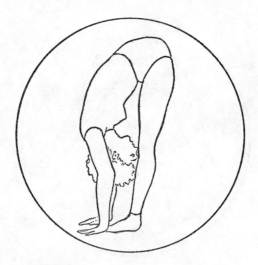

Both feet forward. Knees straight; head to the knees.   (10 seconds.)

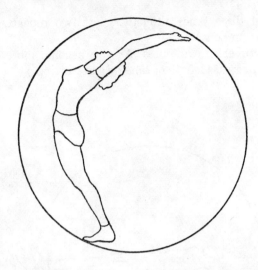

Hook the thumbs; stretch all the way back. (8 seconds.)

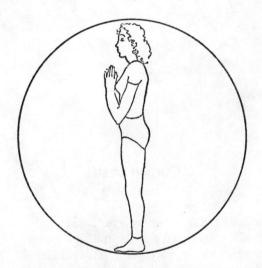

Palms together in front of you. (3 seconds.)
Arms to either side.

(Repeat three times altogether; last two repeats, just say the numbers.)
(Total time: 1.9 minutes. As you become more proficient, decrease length of time on sun worship.)

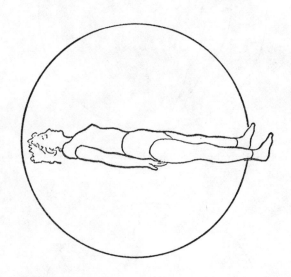

Corpse pose
savasana

Turn around and lie down on your back.
This is called Savasana, corpse pose.
Have the feet a foot apart, palms up, eyes closed.
Just let the body sink down into the floor.

(Total time: 1 minute.)

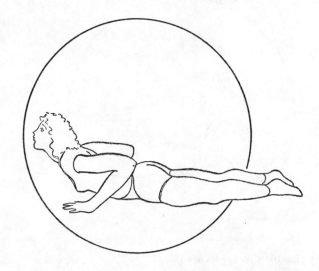

Cobra pose
bhujangasana

Roll over on the stomach.
Put the forehead down on the floor.
Put the palms opposite the shoulders; point the elbows
up toward the ceiling.
Have the arms into the sides.
Palms are down on the floor.
Forehead down on the floor.

This will be cobra pose, Bhujangasana, which is the
seventh pose of the Sun Worship.
You'll be bringing the head, neck, and shoulders up,
looking back; concentrate on the area between the
shoulder blades, stretching the upper part of the spine.

(Preparation: 30 seconds. With more proficiency, decrease preparation time.)

65

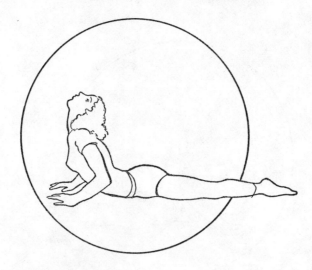

Raise up slowly; look up.
Keep the elbows slightly bent; don't feel that the arms are supporting you; instead, feel the support from the upper spine.
Look back.
Pelvis should be down on the floor.
Keeping the mouth closed, the chin up.

(Up and holding: 40 seconds. With proficiency, increase time.)

Come down slowly, keeping the gaze up.
Now turn the cheek to the side, palms in position, and relax.
Keep the eyes closed.

(Down: 7 seconds. Rest: 10 seconds.)

Let's try it once more, forehead down on the floor.
Raise up slowly.
You should feel that if you took the arms away, you wouldn't fall down.

If you feel that you would, then you've come up too high.
Come down slowly, keeping the chin up.
Relax, put the arms next to your side, cheek to the floor.
Close the eyes.   (Rest: 15 seconds.)

(Repeat: 70 seconds. Cobra pose total time: 2.8 minutes.)

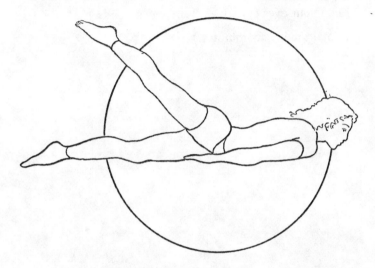

Half-locust pose
ardha salabasana

Now put the arms underneath the stomach; hook the thumbs.
Try to get the elbows as best as possible to touch; have the chin down on the floor.
This will be Ardha Salabasana, half-locust pose.
First we'll be raising the right leg, then the left.
Remember to keep the knee straight and the pelvis down on the floor.

(Preparation: 30 seconds. Decrease with proficiency)

Raise the right leg slowly.   (7 seconds.)
Now slowly bring it down.
Left leg up.   (7 seconds.)
And down.
Right leg up.   (7 seconds.)
And down.
Cheek to the side; take your arms out from underneath the stomach and relax.
Keep your eyes closed.   (Rest: 30 seconds.)

(Total time: 1.5 minutes.)

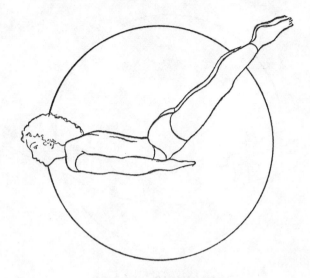

Locust pose
salabasana

Put the arms back underneath the body.
Now we'll try full Salabasana.
If you feel strain in this pose, come down immediately.
Both legs will come up, knees straight, feet together.

(Preparation: 20 seconds. Decrease with practice.)

Come up slowly.
Knees straight; doesn't matter how high you go.

(Up and hold: 15 seconds. Increase with practice.)

Come down slowly.
Cheek to the side and relax.

(Down and relax: 35 seconds.   Locust pose total
time: 1.2 minutes.)
(Keep the same time.)

69

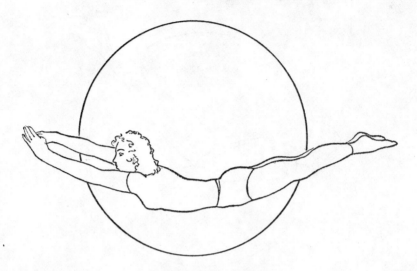

Backward boat pose
poorva navasana

Stretch the arms out in front of you; hook the thumbs together.
Give a good stretch out; this is Poorva Navasana, boat pose.
We'll be raising up on the abdomen, looking out at the fingertips, keeping the feet together.

(Preparation: 30 seconds. Decrease with practice.)

Raise up.
Form a boat; both halves of the body raise up.
Breathe as normally as you can.

(Up and hold: 20 seconds. Increase with practice.)

Come down.
Turn the cheek to the side; keep the arms in position.

(Down and relax: 25 seconds. Keep the same.)

Repeat. Raise up.
And down.
Cheek to the side; arms to the side and relax.

(Repeat and relax: 75 seconds. Boat pose total time: 2.5 minutes.)

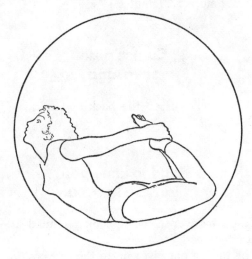

Bow pose
dhanurasana

Everybody grab hold of your ankles.
This is a more advanced pose; if you feel strain, come out of the pose.
Chin down on the floor.
Keep the feet together, and as best as possible, keep the knees together.
This is bow pose, Dhanurasana.

(Preparation: 30 seconds. Decrease in time.)

Keeping the elbows straight, raise up and look back.
And hold.

(Up and hold: 15 seconds. Increase in time.)

And come down and relax.
Let go of the ankles.

(Down and relax: 60 seconds. Hold the same. Bow pose total time: 1.8 minutes.)

Corpse pose
savasana

Everybody roll over on the back and relax. (30 seconds.)

Head to knee pose
janusirshasana

Bring the arms over the head; hook the thumbs.
Feet are together.
We'll be raising ourselves up to the 90° position, keeping the feet down on the floor.

(Preparation: 30 seconds. Decrease in time.)

Come up slowly with control, giving the abdomen a good workout.
Stretch up and look up to the ceiling.
Bring the right leg off at an angle, left heel into the crotch; don't sit on the heel.
Come down to the right foot.

(Coming down: 15 seconds. Keep the same time.)

Look out toward the toe; don't look down at the knee.
Grab hold of the ankle, the bottom of the foot, or the big toe, and pull it like a trigger.
Try to get the bottom of the knee down on the floor.

72

(Holding: 20 seconds. Increase in time.)

Raise up slowly.
Look up; stretch up.
Switch legs.

(Raise up and switch: 15 seconds. Keep the same.)

Stretch up and come down to the left leg.
Don't bounce; come to a steady position and look at the toe.

(Come down and hold: 25 seconds. Increase in time.)

Come up.

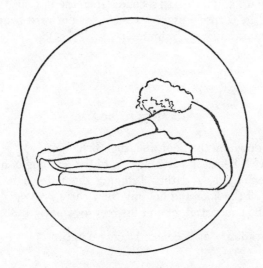

Forward-bending pose
paschimotanasana

Put both feet out in front of you.
Stretch up, hook the thumbs, and come down to the feet.
Look out toward the toes.

(Come up and come down: 25 seconds. Increase time down.)

Stretch up; come up.
Come down to the feet once more.
This is forward-bending pose, Paschimotanasana.
Just breathe easily.
Try to feel as relaxed as possible in the pose.

(Repeat: 25 seconds. Increase in time.)

Raise up.
Now, keeping the back as straight as possible, hooking the thumbs, come down slowly backward.

(Come up and out: 15 seconds. Increase in time.)
(Relax in corpse pose: 30 seconds. Forward-bending pose total time: 3.4 minutes.)

45° leg raises.

Palms down on the floor, feet together.
First we'll be raising the legs up to the 45° angle, holding them there, and then bringing them down to two inches off the floor and holding them there.
Keep the knees straight and the feet together.

(Preparation: 15 seconds. Decrease in time.)

Raise the legs slowly to 45°.
Slowly bring them down to two inches off the floor, and then bring them down to the floor; slowly, with control, and relax.

(Up and down: 30 seconds. Leg raise total time: 45 seconds. Increase in time.)

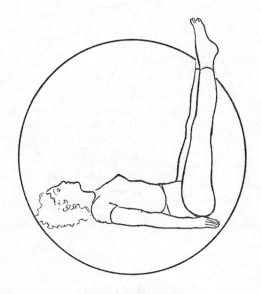

90° leg raises

Now we'll be going up to 90°.
Palms down on the floor, feet together.

(Preparation: 15 seconds. Keep the same.)

Raise the legs up slowly to the 90° angle.
If you can't get them fully up to 90°, you can bend the knees slightly.
Keep the buttocks down on the floor.
Now, with control, bring them down slowly to the floor.

(Up and down: 20 seconds. Increase in time. Total time: 35 seconds.)
Relax in Savasana: 30 seconds.)

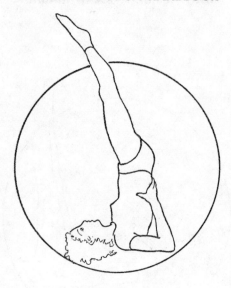

Shoulder stand
sarvangasana

Palms down on the floor again, feet together.
Once more, raise the legs up to 90°.

(90° Raise: 15 seconds. Decrease in time.)

Now we'll go into Sarvangasana, shoulder stand.
Push on the palms; bring the legs over the head.
Support the lower back with palms, and raise the legs
up so that they are perpendicular to the floor.

(Up into pose: 7 seconds. Keep the same.)

Concentrate on the thyroid gland, which is right opposite the chin at the base of the throat.
Keep your eyes closed.

Try to feel the body is as relaxed as possible.
If any tension develops in the feet, or the legs, just give
the toes a wiggle.
Feet should be absolutely free from tension.
Try not to swallow, cough, sneeze, or talk, because of
the very constricted position that the throat is in.
If you must come out of the pose, come out with con-
trol.

(Hold pose: 30 seconds. Increase in time.)

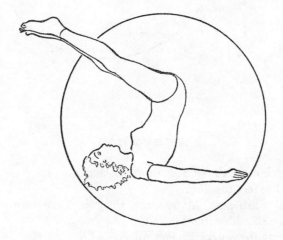

Start to slowly come out of the pose.
Keep the knees straight, put the palms down on the
floor, when you find your balancing point.
And then, with control, bring the buttocks to the floor.
And then, slowly, keeping the legs straight, bring them
to the floor with control.
And then immediately come to corpse pose and relax.

(Come down: 20 seconds. Relax: 60 seconds. Total
time: 2.2 minutes.)

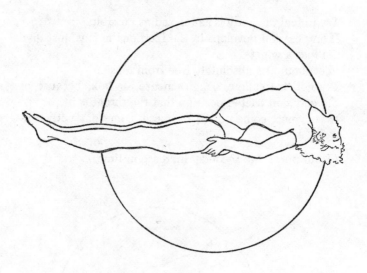

Fish pose
matsyasana

Grab hold of the outside of the buttocks.
Put the feet together.
This is fish pose, Matsyasana, the complementary pose
to the shoulder stand.
Raising the head with control, come up.
Keep the feet down on the floor.

(Preparation and coming up: 30 seconds. Decrease in
time.)

Tilt the head back, placing the crown of the head down
on the floor, arching the back well.
Breathe deeply, keeping the mouth closed.
Again, concentrate on the thyroid gland.

(Holding: 30 seconds. Increase in time.)

Raise up.
Bring the head down slowly. (10 seconds. Decrease slightly.)

(Relax: 30 seconds. Total time: 1.6 minutes.)

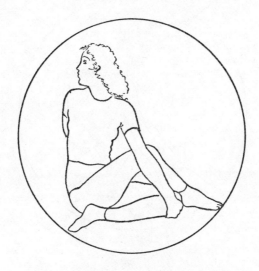

Spinal twist
ardha matsyendrasana

Sit up and turn around. We will prepare for spinal twist.
Bring the knees into the chest.
Put the arms around the knees.
Bring the left leg out.
Put the right leg over the left.
Put the right palm behind you.
Now put the left arm to the right side of the right knee, grabbing hold of the left knee.

(Preparation and twisting to right: 60 seconds. Decrease preparation time. Increase holding time.)

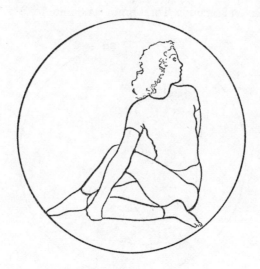

Come back around, back to the preparation pose, knees into the chest, arms around the legs.
Now bring the right leg out.
Put the left leg over.
Put the left palm behind you.
Bring the right arm to the left side of the left knee, grabbing hold of the right knee.
Give a good twist to the left. If you feel a pop in the spine, that's a release of tension in the vertebrae.

(Twisting to left: 60 seconds. Increase holding time.)

Come back to preparation pose.

(Total time: 2 minutes.)

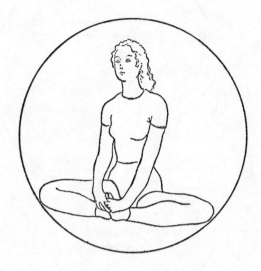

Gentle pose
badrasana

Bring the soles of the feet together.
Grab hold of the toes, and bring the heels into the perineum as much as possible.
You can use the elbows to bring the knees down to the floor, or you can just let them hang naturally.
This is called Badrasana.
Try to sit up with as straight a back as possible.
If you have the heels into the perinium as much as possible, you can try to bend over and bring the chin to the floor.

(Full pose time: 1 minute. Keep the same time.)

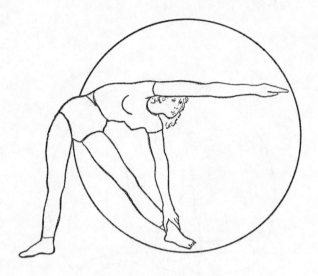

Triangle pose
trikonasana

Everyone stand up.
Put the arms up to the sides.
Feet should be about a foot apart.
The right palm is down; the left palm is up.
This is Trikonasana, triangle pose.
Now bringing the right palm down to the leg, below the right knee, look up to the left arm.
And then bring the left arm in line with the ear, and look out to the left palm.
Try to keep the spine as straight as possible.
Come up.
Now the left palm down, right palm up.
Come down to the left.
Left arm touching the left knee, right arm in line with the right ear.
Keep the elbow straight.
And come up.

Come down to the right.
Come up, and down to the left.
Come up, and arms down.

(Full pose time: 2 minutes. Increase in time.)

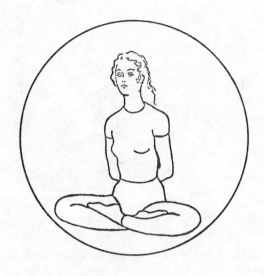

Yogic seal
yoga mudra

Sit down on the floor, legs comfortably crossed.
Put the arms behind the back, right palm grabbing hold
of the left wrist.
Close the eyes.

(Preparation time: 20 seconds. Decrease time.)

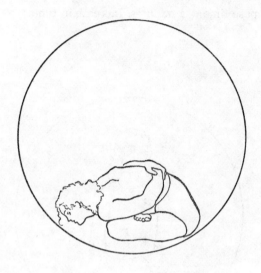

Now come down, over the legs; have the back straight, chin out.

This is yoga mudra.

Keep the arms on the lower back.

Just relax in the pose.

Keep the eyes closed.

Try and have the buttocks resting on the floor.

(Coming down and holding: 45 seconds. Increase in time.)

Turn around, lie on your back, get ready for deep relaxation.

(Full pose time: 1.6 minutes.)

Deep relaxation

Just let the body sink down into the floor.
Bring the attention down to the legs.
Tighten up the right leg.
Squeeze it as much as you can; curl the toes.
Tense it up.
Raise it a few inches off the floor.
When I say relax, let it drop to the floor, as if all the life
had gone out of it, so you can hear a thud on the
floor. (Pause 5 seconds.)
Relax.
Roll it from right to left, and forget about it.

(Right leg: 30 seconds.)

Now tense up the left leg.
Tighten it up.
Squeeze the toes of the left foot.
Squeeze it; raise it a few inches off the floor.
Squeeze it; squeeze it. (Pause 5 seconds.)
Relax.
Roll it from the right to the left, and forget about it.

(Left leg: 30 seconds.)

Tighten up the right arm.
Stretch the fingers out first, then tighten them up.
Squeeze the hand into a fist.
Raise the arm up a few inches off the floor.
Squeeze it. (Pause 5 seconds.)
Relax.
Give it a roll from the right to the left, and forget about
it.

(Right arm: 30 seconds.)

Now tighten up the left arm.
Stretch the hand out, fingers out.
Squeeze it into a fist.
Raise the arm up a few inches off the floor.
Tense it; tighten it up.   (Pause 5 seconds.)
Relax.
Give it a roll from the right to the left, and forget about it.

(Left arm: 30 seconds.)

Now squeeze the buttocks together, draw the anus muscles upward.
Tighten them.
Squeeze.   (Pause 5 seconds.)
Relax.

(Buttocks: 15 seconds.)

Now take a deep breath.
Blow up the abdomen.
Hold the breath in; blow up the abdomen like a big balloon.
When I say release, let the air come gushing out through the mouth in one complete breath.
Tighten up the abdomen.
Tighten it.   (Pause 5 seconds.)
Release.

(Abdomen: 20 seconds.)

Take a deep breath and blow up the lungs the same way.
Hold the air in.
Tighten up the muscles.
Tighten them.   (Pause 5 seconds.)
Release.

(Lungs: 20 seconds.)

Now squeeze the shoulders together.
Try to get the shoulder blades to meet.
Squeeze them.   (Pause 5 seconds.)
Relax.
Give the head a roll from the right to the left and back again.

(Shoulders: 15 seconds.)

Now squeeze the facial muscles.
Press the lips, cheeks, chin, eyes, brows, forehead, all in toward the nose.
Press them in as tight as you can.
Really make an ugly face.
Squeeze, as hard as you can.
Now open up the mouth and stretch out the tongue.
Try to wrinkle up the forehead, keeping the eyes closed.
Stretch the cheeks, the whole face.
Give it a good stretch.
Now tighten once more, all into the nose.
Really squeeze them.
Tighten them.
Relax.

(Face: 30 seconds.)

Now let's come down to the feet again.
We'll work our way slowly up toward the head.
Check out the body for any remaining tension.
Check out the feet.
Keep the body completely still.
Just feel it from the inside.
Check out the ankles and the legs.   (Pause.)
Knees.   (Pause.)
Thighs.   (Pause.)
Check out the hands, wrists, forearms.   (Pause.)
Keep them still; just feel them from the inside.

Keep them down on the floor.
Elbows and upper arms.   (Pause.)
Check out the buttocks.   (Pause.)
The abdomen.   (Pause.)
Lungs.   (Pause.)
Shoulders.   (Pause.)
Neck, face.   (Pause.)
Feel the body completely relaxed.
Just feel it seep down into the floor.
Feel it get lighter, almost as if it could float.

(Body check-out: 2 minutes.)

(Long pause. Body meditation: 3 minutes.)

Bring the attention to the breath.
Just watch the breath, going in and going out.
Don't try to control it; just watch it.

(Breath meditation: 3 minutes.)

Now bring your attention to the mind and the thoughts
within your mind.
Witness the thoughts, and try your best not to become
attached to your thoughts and fall into thinking.
Just watch them. Witness them.   (Pause.)

(Mind Meditation: 3 minutes.)

Now slowly bring your attention back to the breath.
(Pause.)

(Return 1:   45 seconds.)

Now start to feel the body.
Start at the top of your head.
Feel the physical sensations returning to the face,
mouth, shoulders.
The chest, lungs, and the abdomen.
Feel the legs and the arms.

Give the arms a roll and the legs a roll.
Now get ready to raise up slowly to the seated position.

(Return 2: 1 minute.)

Raise up slowly.
Turn around.
Keep your eyes closed.
Breathe deeply.
Keep the breath to yourself.
Watch the breath go down into the abdomen, fill up the abdomen, then fill up the lungs, and then fill up the chest.
Watch it leave the chest, then the lungs, and then the abdomen. (Pause.)

(Watching the breath: 2 minutes. Total relaxation time: 17.9 minutes.)

Now inhale and chant *OM* three times.

(Total class time: 50 minutes.)

Prana, the tie that binds.

Pranayama all too often has been simply defined as breathing exercises. It is, however, a great deal more than that. Pranayama literally means the control of the prana, the vital energy. Sivananda defines prana as the sum of all the forces in nature. Prana is that energy which mobilizes everything in the universe. Human beings are tied to all of creation, most visibly by the pranic connection. When we speak of energy and its interconnecting ties, we are talking about prana. When we speak of the relationship and influence of the stars and moon in our lives, as astrology does, we are really dealing with the pranic influences of these bodies. Einstein's theory of energy, $E=mc^2$, is directly applicable to the understanding of prana. Knowing that everything, including the mind, is interconnected and composed of prana, the yogi attempts to control the mind by controlling one of its manifested forms, the breath. This is how the science of pranayama came about. The student controls the prana, which controls the mind, by controlling his breath. Since everything is regulated by prana, he who holds the reins on prana is a very powerful individual.

Since pranayama is an aid in mind-controlling, it becomes a vital tool in meditation. It is advisable that pranayama is practiced before meditation, for it sets the mind into a state of alertness by both focusing and calming it. In addition, it cleans and strengthens the inner nerve fibers, the "nadis." (See preceding section.) This is an essential process because it prepares and readies the aspirant for a rise in his energy level, which increases as a result of the meditative practices.

The pranayamas.

It is cogent to our present discussion to study, in some depth, particular pranayamas. They are deerghaswasam, deep breathing; kapalabhati, skull shining; and nadi suddhi.

Deep breathing is literally the taking in of a deep breath large enough to fill the abdomen, lungs, and chest, in that order. You then proceed to exhale in the reverse order: first the chest, then the lungs, and lastly the abdomen. In performing deerghaswasam, you should experience the sensation of moving energy, traveling and filling your body from the lower portions on upward. In exhaling, you release the energy from your head first, and then gradually from the rest of your body. If you think of the process of filling up and emptying a glass of water, I think you will find it quite easy to visualize the practice. Deep breathing provides three functions: it strengthens the nadis, and it energizes and revitalizes the system. Deerghaswasam is a very portable exercise; it can be practiced anywhere at any time; you can even do this pranayama when you have a few spare minutes at work. People do deerghaswasam naturally, particularly during the moments of tension or crisis. Deep breathing brings the system back to a normal level, or in other words, it "calms you down."

Kapalabhati, or skull shining, is a practice in which the student breathes rapidly and expulsively. This process energizes the entire system. You perform this pranayama in the following manner: breathe in slowly, filling up the abdomen with air; then exhale quickly. Repeat this procedure four, ten, or twelve times. It is important to remember to breathe in and out through your nose and, at all times, to keep your mouth completely shut. You must always hold your head, neck, and shoulders completely still. You will find, as you become more adept at this practice, that the only thing moving back and forth will be the abdomen. In the beginning it may be helpful to have someone stand and hold your shoulders from behind; this will act as a check on any additional body movements. What will this pranayama do for the system? It will, as I stated previously, energize the body. This increase in energy will, in turn, strengthen the nadis. The rise in energy will be manifested in a physical manner. After inhaling and exhaling a number of times in succession, there will be a rise in the body's heat; your brow may feel a little warm. This is a natural occurrence in kapalabhati; it cleanses the nadis and the entire system through the heat that is generated by the energy increase. A possible side effect of kapalabhati is a slight faintness or weakness. If this occurs, simply lie down in the corpse pose until the feeling passes. Don't be troubled by this; it disappears in a matter of minutes.

The third pranayama is nadi suddhi, or alternate breathing. This practice helps in calming both the mind and the rest of the system. It regulates the two main currents of the body, thus decreasing tension and supporting good health and is usually done prior to meditation.

Normal breathing.

Learning to breathe properly is important for all of the above practices, as well as for your general well-being. Here are a few rules to follow for performing this basic function of life. First and foremost, you should breathe through the nose, not the mouth. Frequently, people develop the habit of mouth-breathing, out of the original necessity to do so when they have colds or allergies, and their nasal passages are clogged. However, the mouth is an auxiliary breath passage, not the main one of the system: the latter designation belongs to the nose for some very primary biological reasons. The nose warms and cleans the incoming air, filtering out the dust particles as they pass through the small hairs lining the interior of the nose. The mouth, however, sends the air, unfiltered and cold, directly to the lungs; a speedy but not very clean nor warm process. The second basic rule of normal breathing concerns itself with the passage of the air into the rest of the body, after it has entered the nose. For this we should use deergaswasam as an example of proper breathing: inhale, abdomen first, lungs second and chest third; exhale, chest first, lungs second, abdomen third. Nose breathing and deep breathing (or abdominal breathing) will utilize the air taken in to its maximum. Becoming aware of our bodily functions, and using them to their fullest potential, is what yoga is about. A further discussion of pranayama can be found in the Raja Yoga section.

Diet.

It is now appropriate for us to discuss another substance our bodies need for survival, food. There are many strange and bizarre ideas currently being sold to the American people on this subject. Some of them are so peculiar and outlandish that they end up providing you with nothing more healthy than a strong and powerful case of indigestion. You've probably heard the proverbial question, "Do you eat to live or live to eat?" This is frequently asked somewhat derisively of the obese or compulsive eater. Lately it has been aptly directed toward those who are extremely, if not overly, concerned with the type of foodstuff they consume. The main guideline to any diet should be sensible eating; in particular, eating in moderation. Extremes in deprivation or overindulgence are to be avoided. Yogis believe that the stomach should be half full with food, a quarter full with liquid, and the remaining quarter filled with air. It often takes many years of practice, and trial and error, to reach this level of moderation. The tragedy is that people have become so preoccupied with what they are putting into their stomachs that they fail to realize what is or isn't a sufficient and comfortable amount for their bodies. Make no mistake, a good, balanced diet is important; however, what is "good" and "balanced" for one person may not be so for another. Thus, though I will be speaking of vegetarianism, I nevertheless know and acknowledge that a balanced diet can successfully be maintained by eating flesh. It is unfortunate that most people do not hold a similar opinion of vegetarian diets. For, the real judge of what food is good for you is your body. If it responds favorably to the diet, it is good for you; if not, it is bad. This obviously takes some experimentation on your part. I do believe that the majority of the people in this country could survive quite nicely on a vegetarian diet. In the same breath I also acknowledge that there are people who cannot; and it would be grossly unfair for anyone to insist that they live on such a diet.

Yogic vegetarianism.

Why do yoga practitioners become vegetarians? The reasons are many. The most important one is stated in the maxim, "You are what you eat." Translated, this could mean: if you eat good food, you will be healthy; if you don't eat good food, you won't be healthy. For yogis, its definition is slightly different, more intricately connected to nature and the nature of the mind. Yogis separate nature into three attributes. Things are characterized as rajas, tamas, or sattwa. Tamas means lethargic, slow, dark, and full of inertia. Rajas is active, passionate, and fiery. And sattwa is balance, clarity, and light. All things in nature can be categorized as a mixture of these three principles. Rarely will you ever find anything wholly tamasic, wholly rajasic, or wholly sattwic. Sometimes we fall into tamas; in fact every night's sleep is an example of it. There are times when we are active, passionate, stimulated; and there are times we are particularly clear-witted, concise, balanced. Yogis, a long time ago, became aware that certain foods affect the mind and body, producing these various states. Westerners are aware of this too, in a limited degree. They know alcohol gets you sloppy or tamasic, and coffee makes you feel pepped up, or rajasic. They also know changing one's environment can alter one's mental attitude. Going to the city can be very rajasic; visiting one's relatives, very tamasic; riding through the country, very sattwic. What one eats is also important in the context of the three gunas: rajas, tamas, and sattwa. In relation to the three gunas, meat is classified as rajasic. It affects the mind by making it overactive and stimulated. Since the yogis were looking for foods to make the mind calm and clear, meat was avoided because of its detrimental influences not only on the body but on the mind as well. Yogis have always viewed food in regard to its effects upon the mind. Their primary desire is to maintain a high level of clarity and calmness; therefore, in choosing foods, they tend to pick those predominately sattwic. That is why you almost never find a traditional yogi eating meat, smoking tobacco, or drinking alcoholic beverages. These substances are abstained from because they produce rajasic and tamasic tendencies within the mind. But, as you saw in the story about Shankaracharya, there are some teachers who can absorb these substances into their systems without any ill effects. They stand unshaken in their state because they are so totally and fully rooted in their consciousness and self-awareness. It is difficult sometimes to discern whether a particular teacher is a true guru, especially if the teacher partakes of meat, liquor, or tobacco. Yet you should not judge prematurely; he or she may very well be a fully evolved spiritual being. Of course, the opposite is equally possible too. For the student, the issue is almost cut and dry. Unless the teacher instructs otherwise, most students in the traditional yogic practices are forbidden to indulge in rajasic or tamasic foods or substances. Most yogis are vegetarians because fruits, vegetables, and grains are sattwic. However, even vegetables and grains can become tamasic if they are inaccurately mixed, cooked, or eaten in large quantities. Becoming a vegetarian does not necessarily mean that one will be sattwic. It is an important step, but one that must be combined with other practices to produce a sattwic individual.

Vegetarianism for health.

Yogis are also vegetarians because they believe it is healthy. They feel that meat, tobacco, and alcohol produce toxins in the system, which in turn adversely affect the mind. Yogis practice fasting for the specific reason of releasing and ridding the system of these toxins. Often my teacher has spoken about the "ine" family: nicotine, purine, and caffeine; substances which are found in tobacco, meat, and coffee, respectively. Through fasting, these toxic elements are removed. I don't think we have to go into the harmful effects of smoking here; numerous scientific studies have more than amply exposed its dangers. The caffeine found in coffee (and in many of our soft drinks) has been reported to have detrimental effects not only on the nervous system but the heart and kidneys as well. Meat also has been coming under scrutiny. For years it has been known that people with a tendency toward gallstones and kidney stones should limit their intake of meat products. Now it has been discovered that poultry is often injected with hormones to increase the growth rate. Even more important for today's overpopulated world is the fact that the grain grown as feed to fatten livestock is using land that could yield more primary vegetable protein than the animal protein gotten from animals. Thus, we are getting less from more, rather than more from less. Now vegetarianism not only means a healthful way of living but an ecologically sound one as well. In view of the above facts, it is distressing to hear our officials refer to the concept of triage as a solution to the world's problems. Is it really necessary for one third of the world's population to starve so that the other two thirds can live? This solution is particularly upsetting when you consider the inordinate amount of meat and grain that is consumed yearly in this country.

Vegetarianism for ethical reasons.

The final reason for yogis to be vegetarians is linked to their ethical teachings. In raja yoga, ahimsa is an important part of the yamas, or the moral abstentions in the raja yoga eightfold path. (See Mind Work.) Ahimsa means non-injury to any other conscious being, and that includes animals. In California I saw a bumper sticker that summed it up quite well: "If you love animals, why eat them?"

I have always thought that more people would become vegetarians if they had to kill their own meat. Now people feel far removed from the killing process, when they go to their supermarket and pick up a nice, neat, plastic-covered package of meat.

We all decry the terrible barbaric way that many people were systematically slaughtered in the concentration camps of World War II. Can we not see the same treatment toward helpless, dumb animals that can feel pain and love just as we can? America has been sold a bill of goods by the cattle industry. They tell us that meat is an absolute necessity, and all sectors of society, from the AMA to the institutions of higher learning to the housewife, gladly toe the line and continue to pay higher prices for their meat. Last year, when the cattlemen were not getting enough money for their calves, they promptly shot them and buried them in a ditch. This was in the middle of the worst world food crisis in modern history. Cattlemen seem to be motivated by greed, and because of it, more meat is consumed in America than elsewhere.

Food fetishes and food fascists.

In talking about vegetarianism, it is important to mention how food can become a personal "trip" or crusade, especially for new converts who are apt to be somewhat militant and ardent in their belief. They have an immediate tendency to inundate you with rules: eat only organically grown foods; don't eat dairy products; eat only raw vegetables; don't eat vegetables at all; eat only fruit. Sometimes you get the express feeling that the only thing they think or concern themselves with is their intake of food. So much nonsense and personal energy is put into the subject and its personal meaning that the practitioners have little time or energy to devote to other areas of their lives. Food becomes an all-consuming passion to them, and this is directly at odds with the fundamental principles of yoga. Not only should we be moderate in our diet but in our attitudes too. As I said before, not everyone should or can eat the same things. Food, like yoga, must be individually suited, and laying "hard and fast" rules on others will not change that fact.

In the beginning, vegetarianism is very experimental. One must try new things to find out what the body likes, what it can tune itself to. The food should basically be light and simple; however, the degree of lightness should be up to the individual's body needs. It is not necessarily true that the lighter you eat, the more spiritual you become. Some people become as attached to the small amounts of food they consume as the big porterhouse-steak eaters are with their large amounts. Remember, the most important thing is to follow the golden middle path. *Make and keep the food simple.* Don't spend long hours preparing elaborate feasts. Certainly, once in a while it is okay; but there is no need to run out and buy a score of vegetarian cookbooks. Vegetarianism is a simple and easy way of eating. If you want a simple meal, slice up some vegetables, place them in a steamer, cook some rice, and in a relatively short time, you've got your dinner. Lunch is simple: some fruit and cottage cheese. For a change of pace, bigger meals can be prepared. And don't think that once you become a vegetarian, you will be eating the same thing one day after another, ad infinitum. There are many more vegetables than there are meats; and they can be prepared in so many interesting and simple ways. Experiment, you will learn the many ways of preparing vegetables quickly. But again, I repeat, save your energy for more important tasks on the spiritual path. Don't let food consume your energies; consume food for energy.

Easing yourself into it.

Years of accumulated meat eating have produced toxins in the system. So when you become a vegetarian, the toxins will come out; the stricter the diet, the more will be eliminated. However, there are possible side effects to a severe dietary change: weakness, dizziness, headaches, and sometimes a whole, dull body pain. Some people experience sharp weight losses or a total lack of energy. Often people interpret this as malnutrition and, after a brief time, abandon vegetarianism and return to meat eating, convinced that their bodies cannot adapt to the new eating habits. All they have really felt is the toxins coming out of their systems and the effects that has on the body. There is a sensible plan in coming off meat, and many people I know have tried it successfully. Probably many more people have done it unconsciously. The plan is simple: slowly reduce and eliminate the types and amount of meat you eat; start by cutting out red meat, then, after a month, try doing without poultry and then fish; and finally, if you so desire, strike eggs from your diet. Be careful, however, when you eliminate meat that you don't substitute carbohydrates for it. Frequently people switch over to pasta to compensate for the heavy feeling they got from eating meat. Other people build their diets heavily around meat substitutes. The latter is very good and acceptable if taken on a temporary basis. However, one has to be careful with this placebo; it may, if indulged in too frequently, hook the practitioner on that secure, heavy feeling as well as add on extra poundage. Meat substitutes are fine as a change-of-pace meal, for they do not contain any meat, but they do contain grains and soybeans, of which too much is not too good. Strict vegetarians of course pooh-pooh them, but there is no need to feel guilty about eating them; just remember to do so in moderation.

The other thing to watch out for when giving up meat is the possible increase in sugar consumption. I've known people, many years off meat products, to become hooked on ice cream. Things like this must be watched, and the body should be checked out on a regular basis to see where these cravings are originating from and why. If you find that you are desiring sugar or other carbohydrates, there are some things that you can do. Eat more protein for a while, trying lentils, tofu (soybean curd), as well as dairy products. Acquaint yourself with whole-wheat noodle products and some of the lighter varieties of grains such as millet, bulgur, and couscous. Try to steer clear of things like bleached white flour; it has little, if no nutritional value. Discipline yourself to eat moderately. You will be hungry and your body will crave more, but after a while, it will get acclimated to your intake. Learn to eat fruit instead of large quantities of ice cream. You don't have to give up the ice cream treats; simply cut down and keep it in moderate amounts.

Fasting.

Fasting, too, is an aid in keeping the body tuned and cleansed. It clears out accumulated toxins from past poor eating habits. There are several ways to fast: the strictest is the water fast. Some militant practitioners insist on drinking either pure spring water or distilled water. I've found, however, plain tap water works as well as spring water in purifying the body. Another fasting technique is to drink raw vegetable juices. You can use the canned variety, or better yet, if you own a juicer, extract the juices from fresh fruits and vegetables. This is not as extreme a fast as water, but it is still very good and healthy for you. This type of fast will also allow you to continue to do your work, while the water fast will quickly deplete your energy. Most people report an actual rise in energy on a juice fast that lasts for several days. There is also a milk fast and a combination fruit-juice-and-fruit fast. Your first fast should be for a reasonable length of time, a day or two at most. It is advisable to start off your fast with an enema or colonic. Your second, third, and fourth fasts should not last longer than two, three, four, or five days; after that, they can last up to two weeks. Always remember why you are fasting. Often people become so enamored with the act of fasting, testing themselves to see how long they can go without eating, that they continue it too long and become debilitated. If you lead an active life, do not become so involved in the fast that you are unable to perform your duties. Fasting is a tool, an aid to cleanse oneself. It is not a way of life. Krishna states in the Bhagavad Gita, "Yoga is not for those that eat too much or fast too much." Often, extreme people become extreme in their yoga practices, and extremism in fasting is a terrible practice at best. Occasionally, if you desire, you can try living on fruit and milk for a week, two weeks, or even longer, without producing any harmful effects. It is a sattwic diet which will help cleanse the body. I recommend this diet in particular for periods spent in seclusion or during the hot summer months.

Special problems.

Some people will have particular problems in cleansing their bodies, especially if they smoke and/or drink alcohol. Yoga follows the belief that the individuals clean themselves by proper diet and practices, resulting in bad habits giving up the individual. Suddenly, one day, he or she will find that there is no longer the desire or need for a cigarette or drink. This, of course, will not happen as suddenly as a finger snap. Rather, the level of craving a smoke or drink diminished gradually, as the effects of having a clean body outweighed the effects of tobacco and alcohol. This doesn't take as long as you might think; actually, it occurs relatively quickly in some individuals. Even if it does take longer than expected, don't be discouraged. If you continue the practices, indeed, the smoking and drinking will give you up. As the toxins are reduced in the body, the desire for tobacco and alcohol will diminish. A craving for cleanliness will replace it. Peace, a result of cleanliness, will replace the disturbed feeling that was present when the toxins ruled the body. When these peaceful feelings are established, there will be no need to rely on cigarettes and alcohol to get past anxious moments. Tranquilizers, too, are a popular crutch which also debilitates the body. However, as you establish the cleansing procedure and practices, and work on perfecting a vegetarian diet, these drug needs will also leave the aspirant.

Special cleansing techniques.

An integral aspect of the Hatha yoga system are the special cleansing techniques which purify various areas of the body. The two major areas cleansed are the nose and the stomach. These areas are of primary significance, for they are vehicles for the important functions of breathing and eating (or digestion). The strength we get from prana, which is received from oxygen and sustenance, directly depends upon the health and cleanliness of the nose and stomach. The cleansing techniques for each are different. They may even be called strange. However, with use, they will lose this aspect and become tools that you will feel honored and privileged to know about. Similar techniques cannot be found in any other physical culture that I know of. I wouldn't be surprised at all that upon scanning this section, you toss the book aside, running away posthaste, convinced that this yoga business is too strange for you. Persevere and bear with me, a full explanation of their usefulness will be forthcoming. I feel it is best to perform these practices in a group. I have found the awkwardness and strangeness of the techniques are lessened when done with other people. It is surprisingly more enjoyable doing them this way, probably because some of the anxieties and resistance are overcome.

Stomach cleansing or water dhauti.

Let us first discuss the stomach-cleansing technique. This is a very simple practice which you've undoubtedly done previously on your own; however, in the past you were probably sick when you did it. It's called vomiting, or literally, throwing up. It occurs naturally when you are sick, or have absorbed some food or substance that is toxic for your body. The peristaltic movement is reversed, and the food comes up from the stomach the way it normally goes down into it. Essentially, this is what we do in stomach cleansing, except we're more deliberate about the procedure. First, we drink five to seven glasses of salted warm water. After doing this, you should have the express feeling that you couldn't possibly drink another drop. When you've reached that point in the practice, there are a number of things you can do. First you jump up and down, shaking the stomach one way and then another. You can pound on the stomach, squat, and move the body to and fro. This procedure helps cleanse the stomach by churning the water around. When you have done that, you can place two fingers in the back of your mouth, tickling the back of your throat while pulling the fingers forward. This will make you gag, and the water will come up just as if you were throwing up. Continue to tickle your throat; the water will soon come out in a steady stream. Don't stop until all of the water is out. Now take a look at the water. In most cases it should be clean, with mucous in it. If there is some blood in the water, it could mean that there is an ulcer forming. After the stomach cleansing, it is a good idea to rest. It is best to abstain from eating for a few hours after the cleansing, and then only drink something mild, like herb tea. Avoid acidic juices or even milk, which has a tendency to produce gastric disturbances.

Nose cleansing.

Next is the nose cleansing. There are two types: water neti (called Jalaneti in Sanskrit) and string neti (Sootraneti). Water neti can be performed several ways. It is commonly done by putting some water in the palm of the hand, closing the left nostril, then bringing the water up to the right nostril and sniffing it in. You then alternate and do the left side. Another way involves using a cup of water or a nose douche. Place the cup at the bottom of one nostril, closing off the other, suck the water in and release it through your mouth. Alternate nostrils, using only small quantities at a time. When using the nose douche, simply tilt your head back and release the stopper; again the water comes out of the mouth. Some people vary this method by using a long-spouted pot. They place the spout in the nostril and pour the water in a constant stream, through the nose and out the mouth. This method works like a siphon; to start, you inhale the water. It then proceeds to flow without additional force. Alternate nostrils. Be careful not to suck the water up into the eustachian tubes, this sometimes leads to earaches. Take the nose cleansing slowly; begin with the hand technique, advance to the cup and then, if you want, to the long-spouted pot. String neti is an even more advanced method of nose cleansing. This is done with an eighteen-inch-long string, one third of which has been rubbed with beeswax. The string should be made of soft cotton. Slowly insert the waxed end into the nose. It will work its way down the nasal passage until it comes out at the back of your throat. Reach into your mouth and pull out the string. You work the whole string through in this manner. The technique takes a bit of practice. Some people have blockages and find it difficult to insert the string; it somehow gets all crumpled up. Others get prolonged attacks of sneezing as soon as they insert the string. These are all common problems and shouldn't dissuade you from trying the technique. Those who have had nasal surgery are the only ones who should definitely avoid the string neti method. If, however, you haven't had surgery and run into a blockage, simply twirl the end of the string around. Occasionally it hits a distended portion of the nostril; twirling the string adds some additional force which helps it pass the obstacle and get down the nasal passage. Once the string reaches the throat, another problem presents itself; how to get it out through the mouth. The difficulty is the string is so far back that reaching for it frequently causes gagging. Instead of grabbing at it haphazardly, insert your index finger and middle finger into the back of your throat and, using a horizontal scissor action, catch the string and pull it out. In the beginning, the area will be very sensitive, so perform the procedure slowly. Once you have gotten one end of the string out of your mouth, you can pull it back and forth from both ends. In the end, you pull the whole length out through your mouth. As always, use the same procedure for the other nostril. As I said before, this technique may well appear strange, but the benefits reaped are exceedingly high. Sinusitis, allergy, and cold sufferers have all profited by this cleansing technique.

Speaking of the neti practice reminds me of a rather amusing incident that occurred some years ago to a group of friends and myself while driving across the country. We planned to stop down in Mexico on our way west, when we realized there would be no place to park our van on the other side of the border. Thus, in the middle of the bridge between Juarez and El Paso, we made a U-turn and came back to the United States. The American border guard was not inclined to believe our story of not having been in Mexico and, after taking a skeptical look at the strange assortment of characters in our vehicle, proceeded to make a general search. He looked through every piece of luggage and brought out the marijuana-sniffing dogs. They missed nothing, not even the hubcaps. Since we were all yogis and didn't use drugs, he found nothing of interest except my neti string. This intrigued him; he thought that it might be used for tying off, so being thorough, he asked me what it was used for. The question drew laughter from my friends, who jokingly urged me to show him what it was all about. I promptly picked it up, inserted it through my nose, and on the bridge between El Paso and Juarez, demonstrated to an incredulous border guard how one made use of a neti string.

Hatha yoga, women, and pregnancy.

The following series of postures (asanas) is designed specifically for the pregnant woman.* This is after any reasonable danger of aborting is over. One should remain aware of the effects the postures are having on the body and avoid those postures which are too strenuous. Only you know when you are putting too much stress on the body, so when you begin practicing the postures, start slowly. Build up to the full set; go slowly. A rule to remember during the pregnancy, the postures, the birth, and motherhood: Take It Easy! Do not neglect normal exercises like walking and climbing up stairs, which are good for the body.

The whole series of postures is slow and meditative and involve relaxation and the use of the breath. They gently stretch and strengthen the body in preparation for a natural and comfortable birth. Between each posture, there is a deep cleansing breath to release any tension or toxins. There should be no need for extended relaxation between postures, but each individual should rest in savasana, corpse pose, whenever she feels the least strain. These cleansing breaths are taken through the nose and blown out through the mouth. This method of breathing is used in preparation for breathing during labor. It has been found most effective in releasing tensions accumulated during the contraction and pushing stages of labor. Another general breathing technique followed throughout is to breathe in on movements in which the chest expands, and out on contractive movements of the chest.

* Women who have already been practicing asanas regularly can continue normal practice for about the first three months, but should leave out the strenuous abdominal exercises. Both new students and regular practitioners can safely begin these special pregnancy asanas in the fourth month of pregnancy.

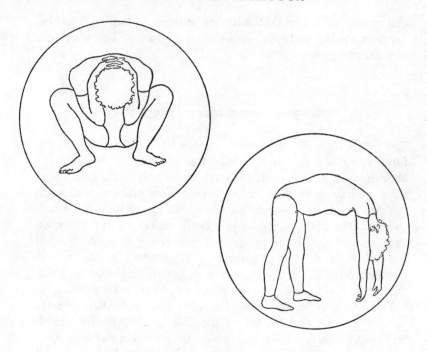

Posture #1
Squatting

Pregnant ladies should squat often, not just during these postures. Squatting strengthens the legs and the perineum for delivery. It is also an excellent position in which to feel comfortable, because it is a most effective position for pushing while in labor. During the postures, the squat should last until heat comes to the legs. While squatting, the back can be given a stretch by pulling the head down, and the legs can be given a stretch by putting pressure on the insides of the knees with the elbows. To get out of the posture, slowly raise the buttocks and let the body hang from the hips for a moment before slowly standing. Take a cleansing breath—a complete inhalation through the nose, filling abdomen, lungs, chest—then exhale through the mouth.

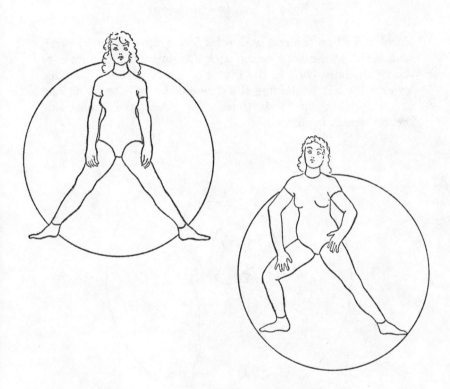

Posture ♯2
Inner-thigh stretch

Stand with the legs comfortably apart. On exhalations, slowly lower alternately to the right and left, raising to the central position in between, on inhalations. Repeat up to six times on each side. Take a cleansing breath. If necessary to relax, do some deep breathing while standing. This pose tones the inner-thigh muscles.

Posture ※ 3
Side stretch in vajrasana

Kneel and sit on the feet with soles facing upward (vajrasana), with hands at the nape of the neck. On an exhalation, lower to the right. Raise back to the center on an inhalation. Exhaling, lower to the left, continuing at a slow meditative pace for as long as comfortable, up to six times each side. Take a cleansing breath; remain in vajrasana.

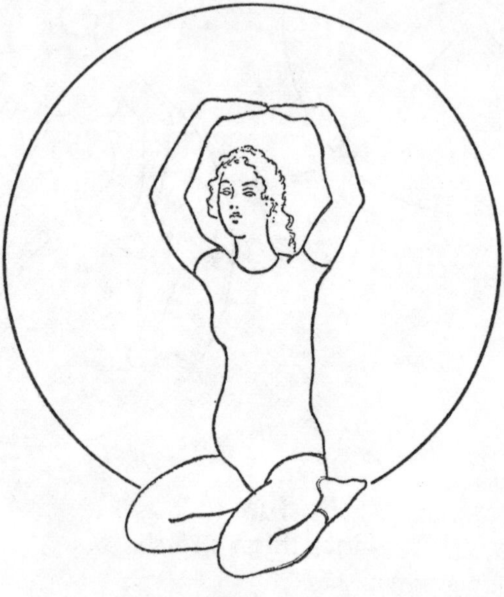

Posture ※4
Diaphragm and inner-thigh stretch

Sit in vajrasana, then spread the knees apart. On an inhalation, stretch arms toward the sky, interlacing the fingers and lifting the diaphragm. Bend forward and relax, with arms overhead, on an exhalation. This stretches the inner-thigh area. Repeat several times. Take a cleansing breath.

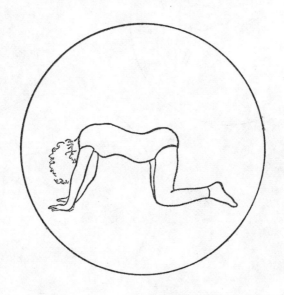

Posture ※ 5
Pelvic rock

The hands and knees are square for a firm base with the body head parallel to the ground. On an inhalation, slowly arch the back, spreading the buttocks, raising the head and neck, keeping the face relaxed. On the exhalation, slowly invert, tucking the pelvis under and lowering the head. Continue alternating up and down as long as comfortable. Gently release posture and take a cleansing breath. Rest in vajrasana. Slowly build up your capacity to fifty times up and down, four or five times a day (upon waking, before nap, after nap, before dinner, before going to

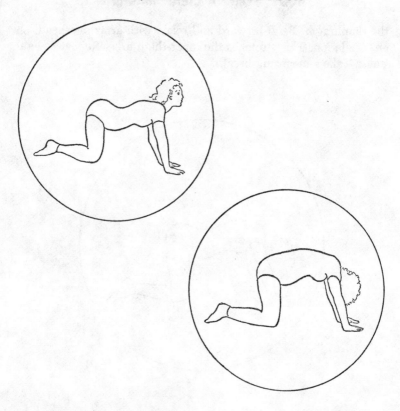

bed). This can be done right up to labor. These poses relieve pressure of the fetus on the nerves and blood vessels of the lower pelvis and upper thighs; and they relieve backache and improve spinal flexibility. Return to all-fours position.

Posture ※ 6
Sideways pelvic rock

Keep the body and head parallel to the ground. Slowly, on an exhalation, stretch to the right. On an inhalation, return to the center, stretching to the left on the next exhalation. Continue as long as comfortable. Take a cleansing breath to tone the waist muscles. Lie on back.

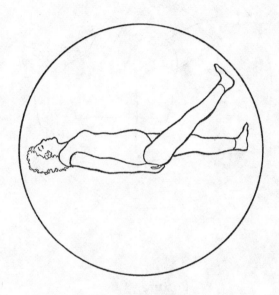

Posture ※ 7
Leg raises

Using the hands to cushion the coccyx bone, slowly raise the legs alternately on exhalations. You can swing them to the sides also. Lower the legs on the inhalations. Continue alternately as long as comfortable. Take a cleansing breath. Benefits: strengthens and tones the abdomen, pelvic and leg muscles and relieves tension, especially leg discomfort.

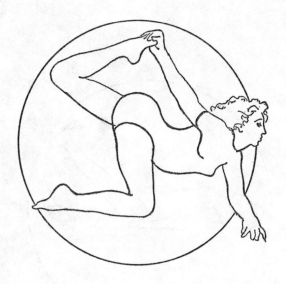

Posture ✳ 8
Raised bow pose

The hands and knees are square for a firm base as in the pelvic
rock. Bring left forearm to the ground, palm flat. Keep right knee
on ground. Raise the left leg and reach back with the right arm.
Grasp the left ankle with the right hand. Distribute the weight of
the body on the left arm and right leg, particularly on the left
elbow. Relax the back and gently raise the left foot, without losing grip. Look up at the ceiling. Slowly come down and reverse
the position, grasping the right ankle with the left hand. Do
three or four times on each side. Lie on back and take a cleansing breath. This pose alleviates back tension.

Posture ⚡ 9
Pubococcygius muscle toner

An important muscle which needs to be toned up is that which surrounds the birth outlet, called the pubococcygius muscle. This exercise can be learned very well while urinating. By stopping the flow of urine, you contract the muscle. This contracting and relaxing of the muscle should be done about three hundred times a day. Take a week or two to build up to that number, which can be done fifty or one hundred at a time, three times a day. This should be done up to labor and again after the birth for a few weeks, until the muscle regains its former tone after being stretched during the birth process.

Breathing Exercise ⚡ 1
Nadi suddhi
Nerve purification

Sitting in a meditative pose, calm the mind. Watch the breath for a minute, using full concentration. Assume the vishnu mudra by making a loose fist with the right hand. Release the last two fingers and thumb. Close the right nostril with the thumb. Without strain, exhale slowly through the left nostril as much air as possible. At the end of this exhalation, slowly, without jerking, begin inhaling through the same left nostril. Take a slow, steady, long, deep breath. During inhalation, first expand the stomach, then the chest. You may raise the collarbones also, and the abdominal muscles will automatically contract slightly as the chest becomes full. This allows the maximum amount of air to go in. Then without holding the breath, gently close off the left nostril with the last two fingers and exhale slowly through the right. Begin the exhalation from the top of the lungs, first contracting the chest and then the abdomen. Then inhale through the right

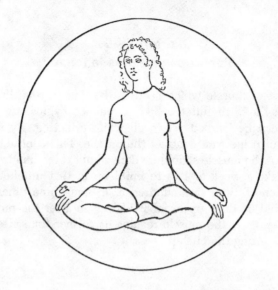

nostril; close and exhale through the left. Continue this for several rounds, gradually building up your capacity. This breathing fills the lungs to capacity and empties them thoroughly. It also calms and purifies the entire nervous system and brings peace to the mind.

Breathing Exercise ✳ 2
Ujjayi
The hissing breath

Sit in a meditative pose. Close the mouth. After a complete exhalation, inhale slowly and evenly through both nostrils, while partially closing the glottis, located at the base of the nasal passage. This is done so that a continuous, soft hissing sound is heard within the head. This sound should be of even pitch and intensity throughout. Avoid all friction in the nose. Inhale, expanding the lungs to capacity. Retain the breath slightly, making sure not to strain. Then, block the right nostril with the thumb and slowly exhale through the left nostril. When done while standing or walking, exhalation can be done through both nostrils. Do not breathe hurriedly or in jerks. The breathing should be done evenly throughout. Even the least strain is to be avoided.

Relaxation Pose

Lie on left side with left leg extended and left arm behind you. Place a pillow under your head. Have right arm bent at elbow, hand palm down next to pillow. Bend right knee and rest it on another pillow. Let abdomen rest comfortably on the floor so that you can feel totally relaxed. (This can also be done on the right side.)

Stay in this position for about ten or fifteen minutes following the postures. Mentally relax the body, part-by-part from the feet to the crown of the head until all the muscles are completely relaxed. Then watch the breath, relaxing even more completely. Then allow the mind to clear, trying to remain an observer to the mind.

After coming out of the relaxation, slowly come to a comfortable cross-legged sitting position. Sit quietly for a few moments before going about your duties.

chapter two – Heart Work, Love Conquers All

Practices of Bhakti yoga, "thought."

Bhakti yoga is the spiritual equivalent to open-heart surgery. It is the path of intense love and devotion. The practice of Bhakti yoga is its own reward. There is no formalized "goal" in this path, as there is with others. Just the constant remembrance and devotion to God bring one closer to the divine. Though there is no "end" in this form of yoga, a bhakti, who is realized, arrives at the same place as other yogis, whose paths seem to be different. A jnani, a raja yogi, and a bhakti all can attain the same high level of communion. The only difference between them is that while the other paths may require strenuous concentration or mental energy, Bhakti does not. Bhakti yoga is considered the easiest path of all the yogas. There are no strenuous physical postures as in Hatha yoga, no long periods of meditation and contemplation as in Raja yoga, and no intellectual exercises as are prevalent in Jnana yoga. In Bhakti yoga all that is needed is a sincere, open heart, and the capacity to love. Unfortunately, novices of Bhakti yoga, after having opened their hearts, often degenerate into cult and sectarian worship. This occurs when the beginners set up a particular teacher or deity as the ultimate god. This type of worship is common in fundamental Christianity; in essence, however, it can exist in only rigid spiritual approaches. A true practitioner of Bhakti yoga, though, elevates himself from the more physical forms of worship, to the supreme, unmanifested form of spirit. A true bhakti may start on an actual form, a deity or teacher, and gradually, through love and devotion to this particular idea or personality, work through the surface form to arrive at its inner essence. For a bhakti, realizing this inner essence means that you have attained the knowledge that love is the binding force of the universe.

Devotion of lower forms.

It is usually not advisable, nor even possible, for a beginning bhakti to start off his or her worship with the supreme form (the unmanifested spirit), for the simple reason that it is very difficult to grab hold of. It is something like trying to hold a bar of soap in the shower, the harder you grasp for it, the more it slips away. Teachers frequently advise aspirants to begin with a deity, an idol, or an image that appeals to them and reflects their own image of what is good and pure. This deity or idol is taken as a substitute for the Absolute, or more precisely as a vehicle to the Absolute. I reiterate, *It is a vehicle to the Absolute, not the Absolute itself.* Degeneration begins when the vehicle stops being a vehicle to the aspirant and becomes the real thing. This is a frequent cause for many Westerners' rejection of this form of yoga. Often, elaborate rationales are woven by both guru and disciple for maintaining that a particular deity is the Absolute, rather than a substitute. Without specifying, one doesn't have to look too deeply to see this form of fundamentalism in many spiritual practices; be it a product of Eastern or Western culture. In certain Bhakti yoga spiritual practices, devotees worship the images of dead saints or martyrs and teachers, not as substitutions but as the personification of God. These deities are not seen as models of godlike people but, by some, as gods themselves. Jewish leaders fear this occurring among their followers. The standards of Judaism are based in its ethics and social laws, rather than personalities. The laws are worshiped not necessarily because they are guideposts, but rather because they believe the laws to be given to the people from God. The laws, in turn, are rigidly followed, even though many have lost their purpose in modern society. However, since the fundamental approach and the rigidness of the devotees are so strong, the laws are still perpetuated. Literalness and the pursuit of the spirit often work at cross purposes to the desired goal.

Chosen deity, ishta devata.

The devotee's innermost aspirations are reflected in the model he chooses. If you have a renunciate's temperament, Lord Siva, who sits absorbed in contemplation on top of Mount Kailash, will appeal to you; if you have a compassionate disposition, you will be drawn to Lord Jesus; if you are musically and intellectually inclined, goddess Saraswati will be your personal deity. The deity reflects an aspect of the absolute. It cuts down the power of the absolute, enabling the devotee to grasp it on a smaller, more personal scale. The disciple worships one aspect of the absolute, not in denial of the other many aspects but in recognition of that particular one he best reflects. Remember, to deny the other aspects is essentially denying the whole thing. That is why blind, fundamental worship is the height of ignorance. However, for the devotee to become established in his practices, and isolated from the attraction of other spiritual disciplines, he must fence himself off from the allures of other paths, as well as from the worldly life. Like a young tree, the novice needs a protective fence so nothing can come and knock it down. First the tree has to be planted, or in other words, the devotee must decide that this is the spiritual path and aspect that he wants to devote himself to, before the fence goes up. Once that is done, the fence goes up only if the disciple wishes it to be there.

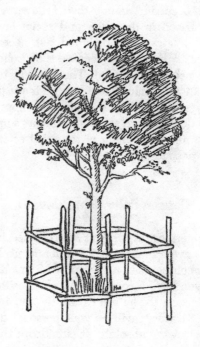

Incarnations.

Incarnation is the act of being manifest in a bodily form. When we speak of incarnations of God, we are talking about those great teachers who, by their presence on this planet, change the very consciousness of the people. They have appeared at crucial moments of crisis throughout history to lead the populace out of darkness, to a higher level of understanding and existence. They may not always affect many people in their own lifetimes, but their influence can usually be felt for subsequent ages. Incarnations manifest as both men and women, to assist us in rediscovering and understanding God. Humans, in their extreme pride, feel that only one human can teach another of something higher. That is why there are stories in the scriptures in which God has appeared before man in the form of an animal, and man, unable to see the godlike quality of the beast, has kicked it out of his home. Even when God arrives in the form of man, man has been blind and ignorant; foolishly wasting his precious time with the god-man, or even, as in the case of Lord Jesus, killing him. There is no doubt that god-men raise the spiritual level on earth by their mere presence, a presence which is felt long after their corporeal beings have departed. I'm dwelling on this subject some because the worship of incarnations forms a very special category of bhakti worship. In the West, we are familiar with one god-man, Lord Jesus. In the East, there are a few others: Buddha, Mohammed, and Krishna. Currently, many spiritual groups are claiming their teachers as bona fide incarnations of god-men and, therefore, true gurus. Without delving into the whole subject of whether or not a teacher is a god-man, suffice it to say that these type of incarnations should withstand the test of time. Whether a teacher is a divine incarnation can best be determined over a perspective of a hundred years or more, where it can clearly be seen if the effect of the teacher has actually increased after his physical demise, or diminished in his physical absence.

There are three basic ways a devotee can use an incarnation in his spiritual practice. The disciple uses both the divine incarnation, and the events surrounding the deity's life, as models for his own existence. The contemplative quality of the Buddha, the compassionate essence of Christ are exemplary guideposts for the aspirant. Devotees can identify, study, and contemplate particular incidents or aspects of the deity's life, such as Christ's crucifixion, or the great realization of Buddha. They are used as models and objects to be reflected upon. The devotee also reads and studies the words of the deity, revering them as the gospel scripture. Herein is where many devotees get stuck. Instead of looking to the scripture as inspiration, they look to it as the only way. If a devotee has a literal mind, he may see only literal truths. It is this pitfall the bhakti must always be on the lookout for. A literal interpretation of the god-man's life and works, when he is alive, should be regarded as God in a man's form. Once he has passed away though, the image or the idol becomes a substitute.

Guru worship.

Many of you by now might be making a mental link between worship of a divine incarnation and guru worship. Indeed, many devotees worship their gurus as divine. And in a sense, a guru is a god-incarnate. He has many of the same aspects of a divine incarnation, and therefore it is quite feasible for a devotee to worship him in a similar fashion. The primary difference is that once a god-man has left his body, his influence increases, whereas when a guru has departed, his influence may not be as great as when he was alive. Devotion to the guru is one of the hardest things to achieve; because, unlike a stone image or a picture or even a passage from the scriptures, he is a living being, always in front of the devotee, always changing and always difficult to pin down. As I've mentioned previously, the guru is a variable creature, varying from friendly to fierce in a matter of moments. This is not the case with a picture or an image, with which one always knows what he has. In a sense, the guru's human form is one of his greatest teachings. Problems usually result for the aspirant when he has difficulty seeing past the guru's personality and form. However, if he has faith, and develops a clear vision to see beyond the surface reality of the teacher, he will discover that that changing surface reality is what drove him inward to worship the unchanging essence of the teacher. No doubt, the transitory and sometimes alluring aspects of the guru's body and personality obscure, from time to time, the aspirant's attempt at a deeper vision of the guru's true nature. But any guru "worth his salt" will see a student who has become attached to these things, and he will work on the student in his task of getting past this particularly vexing attachment. How the guru does this is simple. He simply does nothing, except be himself. This *simple* act is enough to confound the student's mind and blow apart some preconceived notions about the guru. I remember the first time I saw my teacher wearing reflecting sunglasses, or watching TV, or driving his car; each incident blew apart some preconceived notion I had carefully and romantically fostered.

Guru worship may begin as a quite casual affair, sometimes no more important than forming a friendship. Or it might begin as a romantically idealized, guru-disciple relationship, much like a proverbial love story with bells ringing and gongs thundering. One may be, on a simple level, attracted to the guru's personality and message and desire nothing more than an acquaintance of the personal-friendship variety with the guru, or there may be strong feelings right from the beginning. But almost inevitably, one thing is there, an attraction; an attraction to the message which the guru brings and the manner in which he transmits it. These aspects are present from the start of the guru relationship. Gradually this relationship turns from one of a friendly nature, to one of a more serious basis, and as the guru's wisdom becomes manifested to the aspirant, he in turn becomes more devoted. The student will perceive the guru in a truer, clearer light resulting in his seriousness manifesting itself stronger. The disciple consequently feels that it is his dharma, his way of life, to be with this particular teacher. This is an inexplicable feeling that sometimes causes the aspirant to become conflicted. This is especially so when we think we know that marriages are *not* made in heaven, or that we are "the captains of our ships, the masters of our souls." This "inexplicable feeling" is hard for Westerners to accept and realize; though this is actually the situation in a guru-disciple relationship. A disciple feels that *this* guru, his guru, is the one destined for him; it is this particular feeling which binds a disciple to a guru. The aspirant, beginning to sense the guru as a personification of God, slowly and inexorably, starts to surrender to the guru, in symbolic surrender to God. This means the guru takes the devotee and begins to use him in strange ways, illuminating those particular areas that need to be worked on. It is not a matter of the disciple quitting his job, leaving his family, and going off to sit at the master's feet, as it is so often romanticized. The devotee gives up his individual goals and says,

THE MODERN YOGA HANDBOOK

"Guru, thy will be done. Do with me as you wish. I will try to serve you as an instrument; whatever you say, I'll do." Western psychologists find this attitude frightening, that one individual would give himself over so completely to another. But it should not be looked at as some neurotic pattern. The student is giving himself over to the guru, to let the guru work on him. He is trying to realize his own ability to be an instrument of both the guru and God.

Various relations are possible with the guru, as with the Lord. These bhakti, or love relationships, are manifold. The guru can be viewed as friend, father, mother, child, or lover. All the roles are meaningful, with the last one, guru as lover, being the highest and most misunderstood. I cannot repeat too often, the guru is not simply a teacher, he is an object of devotion, as any real deity of a church. It is in this light that these relationships should be viewed.

One must understand that gurus, in many instances, are like children. They are absolutely innocent and virtually uncorrupted. They see the world as God's plaything, and the gurus, in response, play. This is an infectious attitude which the disciples pick up and join in and become part of the play. Indeed, this is one of the most satisfying relationships a disciple can have with a guru. When the guru is in a playful mood, it doesn't matter what he does, the whole world becomes his play-toy. I have seen my teacher toss a Frisbee and even play-act a drunk. At moments like these, the guru becomes "superbly human," and it is also at these times when the disciple is frequently deceived as to the human quality of the guru. Some aspirants, unable to rise above the guru-as-friend relationship, hold on to these human moments. For them, "friend" is an end in itself, and for them the guru obliges. Though guru as friend is a wonderfully loving relationship, it is not the fulfillment of a complete guru-disciple relationship; it is merely an aspect. But part of that unique quality of a guru is his ability to be all things to all people.

The guru as parent is another form of bhakti relationship. In this type of relationship, the guru as father or mother can be as righteous and stern as the archetype parental male, or as compassionate and soothing as the prototype parental female. In these days of women's heightened self-awareness and liberation, these stereotypes of the masculine and feminine role may sound a discordant note. It is not that yogis are sexist, they realize that men can be compassionate, and women stern. In essence, what they are saying is that the absolute woman is compassionate, warm, and loving, and the absolute man is stern and righteous. However, all men are combinations of masculine and feminine characteristics, as are all women. All individuals are a mixture of both. An integrated balance between these two characteristics is ideal. In the current wave of publicity and awareness about homosexuals, these individuals can be seen as people who have a predominance of one sexual component over the other. It becomes ludicrous, therefore, when "normal people" become agitated because of possible contact with homosexuals. What they are expressing is their own fear and, more importantly, their ignorance about their own sexual imbalances. If individuals have had balanced sexual models around them, in their critical developmental periods, their sexual components will mature in a relatively balanced and integrated way. If the early models are not balanced and/or integrated, sexual dysfunction or homosexuality can come about. Homosexuality is an adaptive response to those models. The commonly accepted non-balanced model is the overcompassionate, domineering mother, with an undercompassionate, weak-willed father. But there are others, and, although people may not be homosexuals, they may have serious imbalances which cause them disturbances in their relationships with both sexes. The dependent, the aggressive, the bleeding heart have all had poor models to follow.

A great guru will be a finely balanced integration of both male and female. They do not lock themselves into portraying one role exclusive of another. The guru has realized the masculine as well as the feminine within himself. He is neither man nor woman, but spirit and, because of that, is free to manifest himself in any way that he feels is appropriate. The guru will be a father or mother, depending on the relationship of the disciple to the guru, which is influenced on how the student sees his teacher.

Frequently, the guru's role will change; one may start seeing the guru as father and wind up discovering the mother, or vice versa. The guru feels the need. Very often, aspirants look to the guru for a relationship they never had with their earlier models. Sometimes they look to re-establish poorly formed parental-child relationships with the teacher. The dependent, other-directed child and the rebellious spoiled brat are two types of student that you frequently see. To these students, the guru will give medicine. He may start by giving the student exactly what he or she wants but very soon may switch roles. Suddenly, the dependent student, who was getting motherly compassion with fatherly direction, is now getting motherly scorn with fatherly indifference.

The guru can also be looked upon as a child. This is dependent upon the disciple's closeness to the guru and his ability to form this type of relationship. Often, women form this type of association with their teachers, which the guru permits them to do. It's not that the guru becomes a babbling baby; rather, he appears helpless in the presence of this person. And the person who needs and desires to be helpful, plays out this role with the guru. The guru, in his wisdom, sees this and allows the situation to develop, providing the disciple with the opportunity to work on this kind of relationship. Often, humorous situations result when the guru has this form of relationship with several devotees; it's like a child with ten mothers, each one striving to be the best mother possible. There are sad consequences that develop too; the devotees become so attached to their roles, so enthralled with the closeness of their positions to the guru, that they start to scold the teacher, telling him what he should and should not do. This is another example of students becoming overly attached to the lower form of bhakti worship.

The guru as lover is the most difficult relationship to understand, especially for members of Western society. It is the highest relationship a disciple can have with a guru, truly at the pinnacle of bhakti realization. This is a totally spiritual relationship, having nothing whatsoever to do with physical or sexual love. It occurs on the highest spiritual level, where two souls merge in absolute communion. For this purest and most blissful union to occur, the disciple, himself, must be of a pure heart and a high order of awareness. The disciple is love, the guru is love, and their relationship is love; all are one in this very special union. One of the highest models of this kind of relationship is seen in the Hindu scripture, the Bhagavata Purana. Here we see the story of Krishna, the cowherd boy, and the gopis, the devoted milk maids, and their very special relationship. Krishna, who actually existed, is regarded as a divine incarnation or god-man. The gopis' relationship represent the highest form of bhakti relationship as is illustrated in this parable.

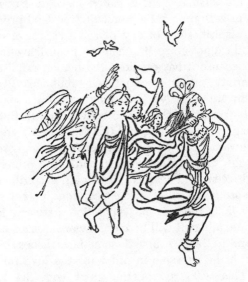

So it was with the blessed gopis; so long as they had lost the sense of their own personal identity and individuality, they were all Krishnas. And when they began again to think of him as the one to be worshiped, then they were gopis. And immediately unto them appeared Krishna, with a smile on his lotus face, clad in yellow robes and adorned with garlands. The veritable conqueror in beauty of the god of Love.

This parable, by the way, also illustrated the concept of Ishwara and what happens to devotees who worship God in that manner.

The worship of Ishwara.

Ishwara is a Hindu term for absolute God in its highest personal aspect. Up until now we have talked about God as a supreme being and God manifested in lower forms. The worship of lower forms should inevitably lead to the higher supreme being. This highest of all personal gods is called Ishwara. But even higher than Ishwara is Brahman, the unmanifested God principle. Brahman is pure spirit, clear of any personal aspect or quality. The human mind cannot grasp Brahman as it can Ishwara. Ishwara is accessible because it has qualities the human mind can conceptualize: eternity, purity, freedom, self-fulfillment. People do not worship Ishwara directly. They may worship a particular god and these higher principles intrinsically within it. But in essence, those principles are Ishwara, and that is who they are really worshiping. Ishwara deals with principles of the highest devotional order. Though they are centered in spirit, the principles can be exemplified, seen, and learned. Brahman is spirit complete; as such, there are no principles, no conceptions, no colorations. And because of that, there is no separation between knower and known. Often, a bhakti will be more a worshiper of Ishwara than of Brahman. In fact, a bhakti sometimes keeps himself from merging with the supreme in order for the love relationship to continue. This was true of the great yogi Sri Ramakrishna Paramahamsa, who as a bhakti, worshiped the Divine Mother in its universal form. For him, the Divine Mother was Ishwara. Ramakrishna often had long conversations with the Divine Mother as if she was right in front of him. Naturally, many people thought him crazy, and in many ways, he was. His craziness was a God-intoxicated craziness, where normal waking reality was less real to him than the reality of the Divine Mother. When an orthodox non-dualistic monk named Totapuri happened upon

Ramakrishna, he began to teach him the way of Advaita (non-dualism). But Ramakrishna, no matter how deeply he meditated, could not get beyond the reality of the Mother. When Ramakrishna went back to Totapuri and told him this, the teacher became angry and picked up a sliver of glass, and pushed it in the space between the student's eyebrows, and told him now to meditate on that. It was then that Ramakrishna was able to cleave in half the image of the Mother during meditation and go on to the supreme realization of Brahman.

Para bhakti, supreme love.

Para bhakti is love without boundaries or support. As a bhakti develops, he or she becomes a lover of all forms and manifestations of the supreme, seeing the face of the Lord in everything and everyone. This is a stage of renunciation; the Lord no longer appears as a physical form, image, or object, the "name" of God lessens in importance. Rather, the devotee senses, through devotion, the force of God resting in all objects, all forms, and all its various names. This realization places the devotee on the path to universal love.

Universal love.

Since the true devotee worships God in everything, universal love, including love for all religious forms, becomes manifested in him. This means that he no longer feels it that necessary to identify with any one particular sect; he is a member of all sects, of all religions, for he feels God in all paths. In extending his spiritual family, the devotee expands his acceptance of all paths, and all spiritual practices; all are as equally valid as his own. All teachers are conveyors of truth, to be respected and revered. And in comparison to the love of God, national pride and patriotic love are specks of dust. Thus, the bhakta is at home anywhere he finds himself, for he can go no place where he does not find God. He is at home everywhere, for everywhere is God's home; he finds himself in any religion, for every religion is God's religion. He is comfortable with all diverse peoples, for all people are God's people and godlike in his image. World unity, universal peace, and love are the only kind of social movements a bhakta would be inclined to support. Anything that would help toward peace and understanding among people would appeal to the bhakta. Small family-friendship arrangements are not considered as important as the larger family of man; universal love permits the bhakta to see every man as part of his family. It is wonderful to see a bhakta with other people; whether an individual believes in God or is a good or bad person, the bhakta treats them all the same. He sees the spirit within them and relates to it; it is that light he sees and speaks to. He sees all men as equals in the eyes of the Lord. Conceptualized thought of right or wrong play no part in his relation with people; for the bhakta communicates with the universal spirit that dwells in all of us. Manifested differences such as sex, color, caste, or age are insignificant to him. The bhakta believes it is his duty and joy to serve all beings without qualification. This great practice, known as Karma yoga, breaks down the individuality that separates man from God. One knows at a glance, these rarest of rare human beings, for to be in their presence is awe-inspiring and profound. Their faces suggest a perpetual light. Even when they are not smiling, a smile seems to be radiating from within. The gaze alone of a realized bhakta is a profound experience. It is so strong and significant that you can hold it in your mind for days, weeks, months, or a lifetime. These individuals are rare, for they understand the very core and inner meaning of Bhakti yoga.

The practices of Bhakti yoga, the word.

There are several practices of Bhakti yoga involving the word, or the use of sound vibration. Foremost among these practices is the repetition of a mantra, called Japa yoga. Japa yoga is the verbal and mental repetition of a mantra. A mantra is a series of sacred syllables. Often these syllables praise or glorify a particular deity. Sometimes they have no inherent logical meaning, merely sounds to produce an inner vibration. Mantras come in all languages, not just Sanskrit, the spiritual language used in many of the yoga scriptures. Examples of Western mantras are the "Hail Mary" of Catholicism, the "Lord Jesus Christ" prayer of the Russian Orthodox, the "Schma Ysroel" of Judaism. In the East, there are the "Nameo renki Kyo" of some Buddhist sects and "Om Mane Padme Hum" specifically of the Tantric Buddhists. The repetition of a mantra is not a yogic practice exclusively. It is used in many spiritual communities around the world.

In this section's discussion of the mantra, I will emphasize and elucidate the connection between the repetition of the mantra and devotion, an alliance which bestows many wonderful spiritual gifts upon the aspirant. There are numerous varieties of mantras: some, and this may sound altogether strange and magical, that bestow beauty, intelligence, wealth; and others, the black-power mantras, which could be used in killing enemies. We will only be concerned with the spiritual variety here.

Motivation and goal should be primary considerations in mantra reciting. The aspirant should never forget why he is saying a mantra. Sometimes, you may lose direction after initiating a mantra repetition; therefore, it is imperative to keep the goal foremost in your mind. There are several simple mantras from Sanskrit that the novice can use without formal initiation by a guru or qualified teacher. Some that I am particularly familiar with are: *"Hari Om," "Om Shanti," "Om Tat Sat,"* and simply the syllable, *"Om."*

A superlative example of the excellent benefits one can derive from saying a mantra are illustrated by the wonderful life of a great teacher, Swami Ramdas, a devotee of the Hindu deity, Lord Rama. He repeated the simple mantra, *"Om Sri Ram, Jaya Ram, Jaya Jaya Ram,"* for seven consecutive years. He performed no other spiritual practice; he simply recited the mantra with devotion and concentration. Because of this single-mindedness, he received full realization, and became known throughout the world as one of India's greatest sages.

Mantras are not prayers, they are praises to the Lord, instruments to open the heart. A prayer is a petition to God; a mantra is a tool of verbal and mental repetition that exposes the inner reality of the self. Mantras have been brought down to the conscious level by yogis from their meditations. They have no real verbal meaning, but their real message is expressed when they are meditated upon. All mantras have a core-seed vibration which is realized when the outer sound vibrations are uttered. This outer sound vibration links with the core-seed vibration within the individual, which ultimately leads to the universal primal sound. The repetition of the mantra should be used in conjuction with devotion, which will keep the mantra on a high level, and orient the aspirant toward the heart center. Thus, if you accept Bhakti yoga as open-heart surgery, you can see that mantras are one of the scalpels. Mantras, like so many aspects of yoga, are highly portable; they can be said anytime, anyplace. All you have to do is close your eyes and repeat the series of syllables. This is the devotee's way of secretly communing with God; a sacred dialogue, so to speak. After the disciple has been consciously saying the mantra for some time, he will occasionally sense a feeling of inexplicable joy. This will be followed by the mantra going on by itself; this is called Ajapa japa, one of the lower forms of communion.

If you're interested in reading further on the devotional qualities of the mantra, I recommend a beautiful narrative, written by an anonymous Orthodox Russian devotee, called *The Way of a Pilgrim*. In it, the pilgrim uses the Lord Jesus's Prayer to attain some very high spiritual insights. The pilgrim walks the length and breadth of Russia, asking spiritual teachers for the inner meaning of the mantra. And what he gathers from them is a very detailed analysis ranging from particular word clarifications to the very manner in which a mantra should be said.

Some practical hints.

If you plan on using a mantra for meditation, there are some helpful hints which can assist you in realizing its full effect. First, when you recite the mantra, pronounce the vowels and "m's" fully for maximum vibrational development. For instance, in the syllable om, you should prolong the letter "m" for the length of time it would take to say "m" several times in succession. Be careful to say the mantra slowly and evenly while verbalizing it. It may take from a few days to a month before you are comfortable doing it. After perfecting the verbalizing aspect of mantra repetition, start using lip movements only, mentally repeating the mantra to yourself. If you find yourself getting confused in saying the mantra mentally, simply go back to vocalization. After you feel comfortable in saying the mantra with lip movement, begin to repeat the mantra mentally, with lips motionless. This is an important stage, for it is here that the mind will wander. It is here also, where two practices interface: Bhakti yoga and Raja yoga. In bringing the mind back to the mantra, we are practicing dharana or concentration. And in our use of the mantra as a devotional tool, we are practicing Bhakti yoga. Once we begin mentally repeating the mantra, the mind will jump around, often freely associating. We must keep bringing the mind back to the awareness that a part of it is still mentally repeating the mantra. When one develops this ability to free the mind from thought associations, by use of the mantra, it becomes a very potent tool. Then, whenever the aspirant feels the mind becoming disturbed, he or she can resort to the practice of japa. There is a cute story that is a variation on a familiar one that illustrates the mind's need for Japa yoga.

Once upon a time (Yes, it's one of those stories!), there was a poor young man who lived by a beach. Everyday he would take a walk along the beach in order to pick up his daily supply of firewood. One day, as he was walking, he met a holy man. He told the holy man what a meager life he had, and asked him if he knew of any way he could better himself. The holy man said that he had a magic oil lamp that contained a wish-granting monster. The only problem was that if the lad ran out of wishes, the monster would devour him. The young man said that wouldn't be a problem since he was so poor, he could keep this monster busy forever. They bid each other good-bye, with the holy man warning if he had any trouble, to call his name three times. The lad said he would, and with that, the holy man seemed to vanish in thin air.

Well, the lad was naturally excited, and he quickly started to rub the lamp. Immediately, the genie popped out. "What is your desire?" he growled. "I want, I want," the lad was so excited, he was stammering. "Quickly," roared the genie, "or I'll eat you." "I want a palace," cried the lad. "It's done," said the genie, pointing to an exquisite marble palace. "I want new clothes," said the lad. "It's done," and the lad was newly arrayed. "I want money, lots of money." "It's done." "Servants, food, women." "It's done." "I want great power," said the lad. "It's done; you are more powerful than anyone else in the world," said the genie. "I want, I want—" The young man could not think of anything else. "Quickly," roared the genie, "I haven't eaten in a hundred years." "I—I—." The young man went completely blank. The genie, seeing this, advanced toward him, his mouth already open and dripping. The lad was petrified, he couldn't think of the holy man's name. He started to run but he tripped, and as he did, he remembered the great man's name. Calling it out three times, the wise man reappeared, none too soon for the genie was right at the lad's heels. "What happened?" asked the holy man. "I couldn't keep him busy enough, sir." "Well, I thought not," and, reaching into his beard, the holy man pulled out the curliest of curly hairs. "Give him this, and ask him to straighten it," said the wise man. The young man did just as he was instructed, and the genie grabbed the hair with all arrogance. The genie first wetted his thumb and index finger and, peering close to the hair, tried to straighten it. But everytime he did, it curled up again. "Now," said the wise man, "whenever you want him, call him and take

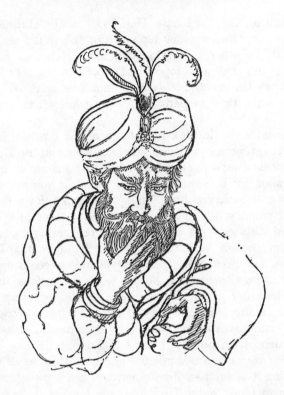

the hair away. When you can't use him anymore, give it back to him."

So it is with the mantra. The mind is like the genie, always ready to devour us. At those moments, give it the mantra to repeat, i.e., the curly-hair theory; when you need it for a task, take the curly hair back and direct it toward the job at hand.

Some further hints.

Next, start slowly and work the mantra into the breath. For example, if you wanted to meditate upon "Hari Om," inhale

"Hari," exhale "Om," or inhale "Hari Om," exhale "Hari Om." Do it either of the two ways that feels comfortable and doesn't force the breath. In other words, breathe, feel its rhythm and rate, then place the mantra on top of it. Don't force the breath to the way you say the mantra. This very important spiritual practice will take some time to perfect, but persevere; it is worth the effort.

Your mantra should be kept both sacred and secret. It is not an advisable practice to inform others of your mantra. Don't use the practices of Japa yoga and meditation as a show or joke. Try to remember, for it is quite important, that, if you demean the practices on which you are pinning your aspirations, they will lose their potency. We have all had the experience of becoming infatuated with someone, and then later on hearing contrary rumors. Even though we initially felt positive about that individual, the rumors clouded our perspective, and we could no longer fully like or trust that person. So it is when we profane our practices, or let other people profane them. By letting other people hear your mantra and possibly demeaning it, you stand the chance of seriously robbing yourself of some much-needed spiritual confidence and power. If the latter occurs, it may become difficult for your continued practice and ultimately result in your abandoning it altogether. Remember, you are a young tree, and you have to fence yourself off from the outside, at least for a while. Furthermore, devotion grows in the quietest place in your heart.

The meditation room.

Once you formally begin your practices, it is important to set up a special room or place for meditation. If you do not have an extra room, you can use a larger closet, a closed-off corner of a room, or a small loftlike platform. The most important part is that it should be away from public view and traffic. This meditation space should be very special to you. Have an altar in it. This can be a simple affair, with pictures of your teacher, or of teachers you admire. Incense burner, candles, and flowers. Keep it neat and clean. Have a white or orange cloth covering the altar. For your seat, you can have an inch board, with a blanket folded over it, and a white towel placed over that. Never go into your meditation room with worldly thoughts; try to feel that this is the purest, most sacred place in the whole world for you. Never put your meditation room on public display.

When you go to meditate, have separate, clean, light, white clothes that will allow you to sit cross-legged comfortably. Leave your shoes outside the room. For as God said to Moses in the desert, "Take off your shoes, for this is holy ground."

Chanting.

This practice, an extension of mantra repetition, can be found in many spiritual settings. Hymns and gospel songs are a form of devotional chanting. The shared communal feeling that is present in group chantings, such as these, raises the consciousness of the participants and fosters a deep spiritual bond within the congregation. Both individuals and groups benefit from chanting. It raises the mind to a high devotional level, preparing it for meditation. Doing it for a few moments prior to saying the mantra in meditation, provides a simple and effective method for channeling excess negative energy toward the proper direction. In the beginning, many people feel a sense of awkwardness and trepidation at the onset of their chanting practice. But I've seen people from varied backgrounds with diverse attitudes, sit down and chant and be wonderfully changed by the experience. For it takes so little effort to do, and it gives so much in response; you need not be a great singer or meditator to feel the warmth and love that comes from chanting simple devotional phrases.

Some practical hints
and further thoughts about chanting.

Chanting is best done in a group, although I've known people to claim they have become very exalted chanting alone in their cars while speeding along on the freeway. Though I have been most familiar with Sanskrit chants, it doesn't mean that other languages are not equally valid to use in singing or chanting. No matter what language you chant in, you should be aware of two aims: a sense of devotional feeling and a high vibrational effect. Chanting can be done with or without musical accompaniment. In certain yogic settings, Indian instruments are frequently used. Harmoniums (hand organs), tablas (drums), and tamburas (stringed drone instruments) are commonplace. However, any group of individuals can gather together, without such instruments, and fully enjoy the benefits of chanting. Chanting can be done in any setting. I've chanted in hospitals, schools, community centers, institutes of yoga instruction, and even at airports!

Though I've said it before, it bears repeating: a proper attitude and a devotional feeling are of primary importance in the practice of chanting. Only with devotional feeling will the maximum effect of chanting be achieved. Singing ability is unimportant, as is a belief in any particular deity or ideology, in experiencing a sense of peace and devotion. And *everyone* is capable of gaining that love and peace. Only shyness and/or pride can stand in your way from doing it. The benefits of chanting are strong and significant ones, and I urge you to seek opportunities among friends and family, or with any spiritual group that may be located in your vicinity. Try to find some common, mutually acceptable spiritual songs to chant on a regular basis. It is an excellent way to bring any group more together, for it provides a means of discovering a true sense of love and real kinship.

Practices of Bhakti yoga, deed.

Puja or worship, the main practice of Bhakti yoga, is seldom seen or known by the casual observer. I am including it here because it is evident that some explanation of this practice is necessary, especially for anyone who is a serious aspirant of Bhakti yoga. Almost all faiths have some physical religious ritual that has a symbolic inner meaning. Yoga is no exception; and in Bhakti yoga, these rituals take their forms from the Hindu religion. Though they are strange and sometimes exotic, they nevertheless relate closely to most known ritual worships. In the Puja, each rite has a specific symbolic inner meaning. Not only the actions, but the mental thoughts that occur in conjunction with them, have inner meanings. Only when an action is combined with proper attitude and feeling does it become complete both externally and internally. The worship, itself, can be performed individually or within a group.

The practice of puja, preparation.

Pujas require a great deal of physical and mental preparation, which is why they perhaps are not often seen or done. Both the physical objects to be used and the mind must be set in readiness for the puja. There is a sense of anticipation in preparing for the puja, likened to the feeling you get prior to the arrival of an important guest. And, after all, that is what the puja is too, the preparation and glorification of an important guest, God. In planning for a puja, you must get the various implements ready and have the worshiper (yourself) in preparedness to receive the spirit, the essence of God. To receive it is to have a most special guest enter your home. The home in the puja is the individual self. It is usual, in preparation for the arrival of an important visitor, to clean the house thoroughly, making sure that the guest room is immaculate and in order. With the same care, the host cleans and attires himself for the occasion. So is it true in preparing for the puja. The devotee showers and wears clean clothes; the articles and room of the puja are set in impeccable order. Once the altar, where the puja is to be performed, is set, the devotee sanctifies the water that will be used during the worship and commences to invoke the spiritual teacher. The worshiper then proceeds to purify himself and the surroundings with the water. After further purification, the devotee invokes the presence of his particular deity, using a physical object—picture, statue, or candle—as a representation of that presence, in which to invest the spirit. The worshiper invokes the presence through the use of his imagination, by sensing and intuiting the spiritual living essence of God. The devotee welcomes the presence as a guest, by offering it a seat, washing its feet (a Hindu custom), and presenting it with some liquid refreshment. Then, as one might offer any guest, you provide facilities for freshening up. Thus, the presence, in the form of the physical object is washed, dressed, and decorated. For example, if the physical representation is a picture, it is washed carefully and dried off. Cloth is placed around it as symbolic clothing, garlands are hung around, and sandlewood paste is applied on the forehead and feet, two sacred areas of the body. Then the formal worship follows: incense is waved, the butter lamp is offered, and food, the fruits of the worshiper's labor, is presented to the deity as an act of self-surrender and sacrifice. After a short interlude, when prayers and chants are offered and it is felt that the presence has accepted the food, the disciple proceeds to the final phase of worship. The camphor light, called arati, is waved, signifying that the worshiper has fulfilled his mission in the divine work and, like the light, will become totally absorbed in blazing enlightenment without leaving a trace of self. Short prayers are offered at the end of the worship, asking support for mistakes committed during the puja, resulting from carelessness of a wandering mind. Subsequently, prayers are offered to God, presenting to the spirit all the worshiper possesses, including any benefits he may have accrued from the puja. And a final prayer is offered to the deity in which the worshiper requests the presence to return back into him. With that, the ceremony is concluded, and some sanctified food is distributed to all who presided at the puja. Cumcum, or holy ash, is passed around. All anoint their foreheads, between the eyebrows, signifying that the spiritual eye—the third eye—has been opened. Pujas are very special events. They can be viewed as odd or strange, but if done properly, and this depends a great deal on the inner attitude of the worshiper, the living presence of God can be felt at these services. Some teachers of spiritual disciplines consider puja to be a low form of worship. However, contrary to this belief, I feel that it is a highly beneficial form of worship for those people that have difficulty conceptualizing a formless God; for it allows you to worship a concretized image of the Absolute in the shape of a statue or picture.

Pujas are ways of meditation too, for they require tremendous concentration and directed single-mindedness. The manner in which the puja is done is equally as important as the inner thoughts of the pujari (worshiper). And as in all practices of Bhakti yoga, puja too can be performed for low spiritual benefits or high ones. Pujaris can be attached to the pictures and the statues, or they can see and experience the high devotional quality of Ishwara in their pujas. It really depends on the level of evolution of the practitioner.

chapter three — Mind Work, Training the Monkey

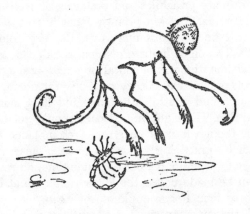

The monkey.

There is an analogy spiritual teachers use to explain how difficult it is to calm the mind. They compare it to an active, hard-to-control, drunken monkey. Its gyrations and movements are uncontrollable: falling, fantasizing, and jumping around constantly. But even worse than that, they say it is like a drunken monkey stung by a scorpion. The mind is not only overactive and falling down in a drunkenlike stupor, but it is also jumping up in repetitious agony. This is the task the spiritual aspirant faces when taking the path of raja yoga. This practice is the science of mental control, for raja yoga slowly and inexorably calms the monkeylike mind. The principles behind it are relatively simple, but difficult to realize. Raja yoga works at stilling the mind by purifying the internal and external aspects of the aspirant, controlling the forces behind the mind and focusing the rays of the mind on one particular object. This object of concentration may be one of several things. It could be a candle flame, your own breath, or a mantra; different schools of yoga use various objects.

The principles and practices of raja yoga are contained in the raja yoga sutras by Patanjali. There are several editions of the sutras, the simplest edition I am familiar with is *How to Know God,* by Christopher Isherwood and Swami Prabhavananda. It covers the primary principles and practices, as well as the various states of realization. My primary focus in this discussion on raja yoga will be on Ashstanga yoga, the eightfold or eight-limbed path. The eight limbs are yama, the don'ts or moral abstentions; niyama, the do's or moral practices; asana, the seat or body control; pranayama, energy control; pratyahara, sense control; dharana, mind control; dhyana, mind flow; and samadhi, mind absorption. The eight-limbed path should not be regarded as a ladder, though it does bear some resemblance to one. An aspirant can be practicing yamas, niyamas, asanas, pranayama, pratyahara, and even dharana at the same time; however, no real progress can be made unless the lower rungs are at least somewhat mastered first. For example, no one can become absorbed in samadhi, the superconscious state, without first being able to practice the moral controls and the energy and sense controls. It is not possible to simply "jump into" the superconscious state. There are no short cuts in yoga; it is a slow, systematic practice. I am naturally suspicious of any school of yoga that claims to know ways of making the process of attaining enlightenment quick and easy. Nothing that is really worth anything can be gained without work. Samadhi cannot be achieved by a few spare moments of meditation, a couple of choice words from the guru, and a parting pat on the head. It is a disservice to yoga and the whole yogic way of life to think this high state is so easily come by.

Yama, the don'ts.

The yamas and niyamas are generally regarded as the yogi's ten commandments. Yama consists of non-killing, honesty, non-stealing, continence, and non-receival of gifts. Any one of these yamas can be a path and used as a guiding force in your life. Unfortunately, these moral codes, as well as the commandments of the Old Testament, are looked at an anachronisms today. These moral codes, for the most part, are not practiced or respected with any regularity or consistency in America, 1975. It appears that Western society has spent the first three quarters of this century overcoming the effects of the Victorian Age. In some areas, it seems that the reaction to the illness is greater than the illness itself. Moral codes are not designed to oppress or repress natural instincts, rather, they are useful guides in channeling and directing them. Instincts left uncontrolled can lead the individual into serious difficulties and disturbances. Once the individual is in a disturbed state, the fabric of society begins to tear; for the individual is the foundation of society, one of the many threads that make up the fabric. For example, the yama of non-killing (ahimsa in Sanskrit) is important to the strength of the thread and the stability of the fabric. In today's society, violent crimes are increasing. And it is evident that acts of violence are, to a degree, extolled, consciously and unconsciously. There are numerous examples where it is illustrated on a one-to-one basis, as well as on a societal level. Not only does regular evening television exhibit a high incidence of violence, but also Saturday morning viewing, which is primarily for children. Play guns have been, and probably will be for some time, a popular plaything for children. Hunting, once an act of subsistence and now a sport, is, through the overzealousness of some individuals, endangering the existence of some species of wildlife. Now even the name of the sport is becoming demeaned. Men go out to small hunting preserves to shoot exotic and domestic animals, in a shooting-gallerylike atmosphere, so that they can mount their victims' heads above their mantels. Well-meaning farmers and ranchers are instrumental, too, in this decimation. In an attempt to maintain their livestock, they have trapped and killed the wolves and coyotes of the prairies, bringing these animals ever closer to the brink of extinction. Insecticides, used to protect our crops and flower beds, are doing more than killing insects; they are also whittling away at the supports of nature's balance. Man must learn to touch the universe and nature with a light hand, or else face the possibility of living alone on a stark and poisoned planet.

Large societal ills start with small, insignificant sores. Petty larceny is such a sore. Good citizens take supplies from their offices, cheat on their income tax, and take advantage of others' mistakes with impunity. These individualized small-scale robberies help create an atmosphere in which larger, socially unacceptable, robberies can occur. We must stop thinking of ourselves as being isolated and realize that we affect the whole society. It is an illusion to believe that because the country is so large and multivarious, people can do as they please and feel safe in the belief that their acts are going unnoticed. The truth is the opposite; things are taken note of, and what one person does not only affects his neighbor, a part of society, but also the whole. This is why moral codes are important. Indeed, I grant you, they have in the past been used as repressive measures on individuals and their development. But today we are ready for a balanced application of firm moral principles. This country, this society, this world and the people in it cry out for this application.

Non-killing, ahimsa. Ahimsa means non-killing or non-injury to any living thing in thought, word, or deed. "Wait a minute," you're probably saying, "in the section on vegetarianism, you came out against killing animals, but not vegetables. Aren't they alive too?" Yes, they are. We now know, through scientific testing, that plants are not only alive but possess rudimentary emotions. Ahimsa is designed to free man from the useless, rampant killing of both vegetable and animal life (which includes, lest we forget, humans too). Yogis try to consume foodstuff that is on the lower levels of the evolutionary consciousness scale. In other words, yogis see living matter in stages of awareness and complexity; the lowest being plant life, higher up non-human animal life, and ultimately the highest conscious animal we know of, *Homo sapiens*. Plants, being lower than animals on the evolutionary scale, were selected for that reason. However, the useless killing of plants and trees is definitely contrary to the principle of ahimsa. Let us remember, too, that ahimsa also deals with the harming of people in word and thought, as well as deed. Many of us go through life without harming a fly, so to speak, but, in fact, through verbal abuse and insensitive thoughts have caused great injury. Hypercriticism and gossipmongering are like throwing darts at a person and sometimes just as injurious.

The purification of an individual, in ahimsa, must begin on the thought level. In yoga, thoughts are considered to be as powerful, if not more so, than actual deeds. What a person thinks is ultimately what he becomes. A person's thoughts affect other aspects of the mind. How the mind is affected will influence the personality, and how the personality is affected will touch one's destiny, and how the destiny is affected will influence one's life. So, thoughts are the foundation blocks of a person's life. If a person has rageful and hostile thoughts, the mind of this individual will possess an overabundance of anger. His personality will be infected by this anger, and it will touch and influence his fortunes, abilities, and relationships. How *these* are affected will consequently alter his life.

Mahatma Gandhi built his political philosophy around ahimsa. He showed how passive resistance could move nations. Only when man has a pure heart and great love, can he resist the anger, hatred, and brutality of his adversaries. Gandhi showed that only a truly fearless and courageous man could practice ahimsa thoroughly. It takes little courage to carry a gun and shoot somebody; it takes a great deal of courage *and* love to stand in front of your fellow man, when he is at his worst, and remain fearless. Martin Luther King, Jr., also took ahimsa and used it to attain great political results. Killing, by pulling the trigger on a gun, is one of the simplest acts a man can perform, but creating a life is an impossible act for him. Why, if man has not created life, does he feel that he has the right to destroy it? Many supposedly God-fearing men wait expectantly for the hunting season so they can take the lives of innocent animals. Many God-fearing men instigate stupid and insipid wars, wasting and destroying the lives of our youngest and healthiest citizens. How long can the earth exist in such a manner? Imagine beings from a more advanced planet landing on earth. They'd probably look at us, shake their heads, and wonder sadly, "Why do these people fight and kill one another? Why do they destroy innocent creatures for nothing more significant than a pandering of their masculinity?" We would certainly seem primitive and brutal to these individuals. If only we could develop our consciousness and see our way through this ludicrous behavior.

Truthfulness, satyam. Speaking the truth is, and has always been, a great moral virtue. Unfortunately, this great virtue is slowly and inexorably being eroded away in contemporary daily life. We see individuals, daily and repetitively, telling small and expedient lies, using those means to get ahead of someone else. This destructive lying has its effects. Why people become shocked when politicians or corporations lie, or look aghast at the duplicity of nations, is beyond me. After all, our own lying, in our own small ways, contributes to this attitude. "Don't tell so-and-so; he doesn't *have* to know" or "Don't be a fool and tell the truth" are attitudes frequently expressed. We must realize that we do not exist in a vacuum, isolated and free from influencing those around us. We know that there is an ecology of nature, but we have yet to realize an ecology of morality. We are unwittingly polluting our moral headwaters, only to discover a much larger crisis downstream.

Truthfulness is one of the most important moral precepts and one of the least understood. There *are* some exceptions to consistently telling the truth, but you must use them judiciously and wisely. If your truth will hurt somebody needlessly, then it is wiser to temper it with a small lie. If your lying will hurt someone, then it's best to speak the truth. If caught in the dilemma of causing pain whether you lie or speak the truth, speak the truth, but always with tenderness and compassion. Lately, it is fashionable for people to form groups for the express purpose of being honest to one another. Unfortunately, these encounter groups usually possess a modicum of tenderness and love, using honesty as a bludgeon, a tool of destruction, wielded out of anger and hate. These cathartic bursts of honesty may be very dramatic, as in Eugene O'Neill's *Long Day's Journey Into Night*, but they don't produce lasting, stable relationships. Speaking the truth, with tenderness, constructs a reservoir of will power, which has a transforming effect on making one a tranquil individual. This often happens in a roundabout way. For example, an individual may run into a situation where it is more expedient to lie than to tell the truth. The person feels guilty and confused in his predicament. He has the proverbial angel on one shoulder, and the devil on the other. Once he has established himself by speaking the truth, there will be neither angel nor devil, just himself with the moral principle of honesty internalized.

Non-stealing, asteya. Non-stealing may be one of those fairly obvious yamas you feel does not necessitate considerable explanation. As we've discussed in ahimsa and satyam, we are basically concerned with these principles as they can be applied in small ways. We know that stealing and robbery go on in covert and overt ways. Petty "rip-offs," like the ones mentioned previously occur so frequently, and are taken for granted by everybody, that they could be considered indigenous to our society. Stealing is symptomatic of deeper problems in America, as is defacing of public property; graffiti on public-transportation conveyances has reached epidemic proportions in some cities. Stealing and defacing, in essence, are one and the same thing. They exhibit a deep sense of alienation from the community-at-large. There is a prevalent feeling of powerlessness and inability to affect one's own destiny. These deviant behaviors are a crying out, a disruptive attempt, to be heard. The thief goes one step beyond the defacer; he is retaliating against society for the maltreatment he believes he has received from it. If stealing was only occurring among the poorer classes, we could partly claim the cause was the result of their disenfranchisement from the rest of society. But stealing and defacing are not only the providence of the low-income classes, they also occur, with some frequency, in the middle classes as well. Individuals do not act as parts of the community-at-large; they feel isolated; nothing binds them to the world outside their cubicles of existence. These deviant attitudes, which reflect a feeling of aloneness, are communicated and learned at the family level. Children see parents take towels from a hotel room, so they in turn see nothing wrong in taking candy from the corner store. This reactive process seems to have no end. Though no one wants to live in a community of thieves, that nevertheless appears to be where we're heading. Non-stealing is a practical moral code that is necessary at this time and for all yoga aspirants.

Continence, brahmacharya. The subject of sexual continence is discussed fully in Part three, chapter two.

Non-receiving of gifts, aparigraha. This is a difficult concept for some people to understand. Let us look at it as a yogi sees it. There are two kinds of gifts one can receive, those given out of love and those given out of duty. Gifts given out of love can never bind you, for they don't demand to be reciprocated. However, what usually happens is that a gift is given out of obligation, not love. It is somebody's birthday or graduation, and the celebrant expects recognition, usually in the form of a present. This attitude is an imposition, ever so slight, but, nevertheless, it is one. All are expected, or even ever so subtly commanded, to "toe" the gift-giving line. An extreme form of this behavior is exemplified by parents of newly married children attending a wedding of their friends' children. What kind of gift should they get? How much did their friends give to *their* children? How much money are they obligated to spend? It sounds gross, but if you think about it, it rings true. The newly married couple in their turn follows through and perpetuates this line of reasoning. Right after the wedding, the bride and groom go through the list of guests, tabulating what each person has given, making sure that everyone has fulfilled his or her gift-giving obligation. The yoga aspirant should always be wary of falling into this kind of relationship. But please don't hesitate to give a gift out of love, for a gift out of love is the most beautiful expression. I have seen a person give a beautiful wildflower with such deep love that a most expensive gift could not compare with it. This is truly a gift, not an obligatory duty. The recipient of such a present knows the gift for what it is, a representation of the giver's deep affections and love.

Niyama, the do's.

Niyamas comprise five aspects: cleanliness, contentment, austerity, study, and self-surrender to the Lord.

Cleanliness, soucha. The old adage "Cleanliness is next to godliness" stands at the center of soucha. Godliness cannot exist in either a filthy body or mind. If the body is dirty, the mind is dirty too, producing a film around the godlike essence of the individual. Romantic literature, which has portrayed the Indian yogi as a semiclad, dirty vagabond, seems to have forgotten or neglected this niyama. The truth is that yogis have *never* forgotten this precept. Most are clean, orderly individuals in command of themselves and their environment. To them, cleanliness is natural, part of their way of life. Back around 1965, when my teacher first came to this country, we were in the midst of the counterculture revolution. For the most part, those of us who came to him were young, free-wheeling, and rather dirty. Soucha was one of the first practices he taught us. Cleanliness of mind, body, and physical environment was impressed upon us. Our lessons in cleanliness took various forms; from repainting and regularly cleaning the yoga institute, to proper food etiquette, to ultimately cleaning up our own life-styles. It seemed rather strict and formal then, but the practice lasted and stood us well through the years. Ignorance is like dirt around the mind. As you clean the outer layers of your environment and body, you are also working out the deep and persistent grime surrounding the mind.

Contentment, santosha. A yogi should experience a feeling of contentment in his everyday existence. This does not mean that he walks around all day with a silly grin on his face. He knows a sense of satisfaction that is born from deep inside the Self. This sense of contentment is absolutely necessary in attaining higher states of consciousness. It is the natural birthright of man to be contented. If an individual is malcontent, all his mental energies will be consumed in disturbing conflicts, leaving little power to pursue further spiritual study. Therefore, the highly neurotic person cannot really successfully practice raja yoga. His personal problems will be too disruptive to the meditative process. In conjunction with this, you should be aware and not expect yoga to solve any deep complex problem that you may have. There are professional people who are trained to help and assist you to work out such problems. Yoga does help people who feel that their lives are unfulfilled in one aspect or another. This, however, is quite different from neurotic personal conflicts. An individual may feel content and unfulfilled at the same time, as if something was missing from his life. Serious aspirants usually try many ways to fill up this void. The neurotic person, unlike the contented but unfulfilled individual, is dealing with the lack of fulfillment in his life, as well as his inability to cope with reality. In order to practice yoga, one must be able to cope with reality well. Contrary to popular belief, yogis do not run away from reality. They, instead, use reality and its harsh lessons as a great teacher. This kind of practice would be impossible for the neurotic individual.

Austerity, tapas. Tapas means fire, and the practices of austerity are designed to burn away the impurities of the mind; but unfortunately there is a great deal of misunderstanding about this point. Austerities don't mean becoming a flagellant or skinny ascetic; neither I nor you should be interested in those cruel, self-inflicted tortures of the Middle Ages. Those forms of austerity were abominations of true spirituality, and they did little in advancing the aspirant. Such austerities as the fakir's practice—lying on a bed of nails, or holding an arm up in the air until it withers, may produce nothing more than a great ego. Austerity must be practiced as well as oriented toward increasing one's understanding. There is an excellent story about an aspirant who decided he was going to practice tapas to learn to walk on water. He asked a great teacher about this practice, and the teacher informed him that he knew nothing about walking on water. "I thought you were a great teacher," the disciple exclaimed. "Well," the guru responded, "some think of me in that way, but, as to your request, I simply do not know how to walk on water."

The disciple left, determined to practice the austerities and learn this miraculous power. For many years he practiced austerities and fasted regularly, until one day he decided to try to attempt the difficult feat. Nearby there was a wide river, which could only be crossed by a ferry boat. With a great deal of concentration and effort, the disciple walked over it to the other side. Excited and exhausted from the effort, he went immediately and told the old teacher of his accomplishment. "Guru," he said hoarsely, "I did it. I learned how to walk on water, and today I crossed the river." "Mmmmmm," the guru sighed, looking at the bedraggled figure, "and how long did it take?" "Only fifteen years." "Fifteen years to cross over the river, and it will only take me five minutes to do the same in a boat. You wasted your time and energy, my son; you should have spent it more wisely and used your austerities for more spiritual purposes."

Tapas works as an internal fire, burning away the gross impurities, the selfish, dark qualities of the ego. For the goal of yoga is to have a healthy ego, not a self-centered one, and we need a strong one to help us function fully in all realms of endeavor. Transcendence of the ego is a goal of yoga, but one does not keep that state forever. Therefore, it is wise to have a healthy, solid ego to return to. Some external tapas, such as fasting and silence, have certain beneficial effects on purifying the gross impurities of the ego. Anyone, according to his circumstance and capacity, can do these tapas. I believe, though, that the real tapas is the taking of pain without returning it. The pain I am referring to is the internal, psychic pain; for example, that which is caused by separation from material objects or possessive relationships. Physical pain may come into play too, when it directly relates to psychic pain. We have all felt the pangs of psychic pain. You set your hopes on something, and "for no reason at all," they are dashed. You expect someone to come visit, and they don't. A sure thing falls through. Psychic pain is part and parcel of everyone's life. There is no way to avoid it, though various means are used to blanket its presence; overindulgence in food or drink, or a heavy drug reliance. Psychic pain acts as an indicator; it tells the individual he is out of harmony, no longer in balance, with his nature. Pain occurs when a person focuses his self on the external world, trying to hold on to and possess a part of it. This destroys the balance of his internal nature. In dealing with this disharmony, one must first accept it; this act quells and subdues the selfish part of the ego, which otherwise would attempt to restore self-respect by transferring the pain to another person, or demanding it by overindulgence. The lesson here is that one must learn to live, and use, pain as a teacher. As you can see, austerity and non-injury are inexorably linked. Physical pain shows the aspirant how transient physical well-being is and why it is important to strive for a deeper reality beyond and beneath the physical realm. Mental pain illustrates the same thing, only this time on the functioning level of the mind. Mental contentment itself is a fleeting thing, though we often fool ourselves into believing that it will last forever. Pain forces us inward, to question, "Why did this happen to me? What did I do? Where did I go wrong?" Swami Sivananda's story about a young man who came to see him exemplifies this inward force. The young man was perplexed and asked him, "Swamiji, you say that all things are good. What good are the mosquitoes?" "Well," the swami responded, "they bite us and therefore show us how transitory life and physical contentment are. We must thank the mosquitoes for shaking us out of our lethargy and showing us there is something more."

Deep personal attachment is usually the cause behind, and the answer to, the eternal question, "Why me?" My teacher has a saying he often uses to emphasize cases of this kind, "You will never get disappointed," he says, "if you don't make any appointments." In not reciprocating pain, you are able to halt the circular process and trace it back to the advent of the pain. It all begins with an attachment, an appointment which you created and maintained. That is why you become disappointed when something comes along to sever you from your attachment. In essence, you alone are the person who seals your doom by attaching. It is so easy to blame other people, circumstances, or even God for failure; but it is ever so hard to search within yourself to find the real reason for the pain. It is selfishness, in its all-consuming presence, that blinds the individual, keeping him ignorant to the cause of the pain and anguish. Only this kind of tapas will work, for it is the only type that will dig deep into the selfishness and ignorance that binds and blinds us.

Study, swadhaya. Yogis have a tradition of disrespect for intellectualism. They believe that books are vehicles of printed knowledge; and wisdom, as such, cannot be learned from them. This, I believe, is true. Wisdom is the process of removing ignorance; this is done by maintaining an open and fully conscious mind throughout your life. Study from the scriptures can give guidance and inspiration, leading to further self-examination. Study can also be used as a form of satsanga. One of an aspirant's primary duties is to actively keep satsanga, or spiritual discussion, in his life. One is not apt to be surrounded by spiritual devotees on the path, so, obviously, the quickest and easiest method of having a spiritual dialogue is to keep a library of spiritual books and readings. Study provides examples of spiritual men and women, whom you can use as guideposts. In reading about these people, their problems, and how they rose above them, you are provided with tangible guidance and inspiration. This allows you to reflect on the teachings of the sages, since the people themselves are, in essence, the teachings. Using the scriptures in this manner can only produce good. Therefore, though study cannot produce wisdom, it can nevertheless lead you to its doorstep.

Self-surrender to God, Ishwara pranidhana. Translated, this term is the act of surrendering the fruits of one's labors to the Lord. "Thy will be done" is the central axiom of Ishwara pranidhana. In order for His will to be done, you must first surrender to God, thus permitting His greater power to take over. Surrender is neither an easy nor quick process. To surrender is to give up, relinquish personal attachments. Most of us would find giving up these attachments difficult, especially when considered in conjunction with the fact that, for the greater part, we are ignorant of what they really are. That is why tapas and self-surrender are so interlocking in aims. In preparation for self-surrender, one should peruse one's life and attachments and mentally begin to sever the latter from the mind. This practice may necessitate constant repetition, but it will, in the end, bear important spiritual results. After you have decided to dedicate yourself to the Lord, take everything you own and mentally set them before yourself for examination. Detach yourself from these articles; they are no longer yours. You are the guardian, not the owner, of the house, car, property, and money, and, as such, receive neither personal power nor prestige from them. Next, take all your friends, relatives, and acquaintances and again mentally place them before you. "You are no different from the rest of humanity. I do not own you and you do not own me. I love you, but beyond the realm of simple obligation, I owe you nothing special." Children too are not to be owned or held in obligation to you. You are their caretaker and that only temporarily. Finally, is the realization that whatever you do, henceforth, is God's work, to be considered great and important, no matter if the task is small or large. Surrender yourself to the divine slowly, bit by bit.

Posture, asana. Asana is the third limb of the eight-limbed path. Asana is the act of keeping a steady or firm meditative posture. This aspect of the raja yoga sutras is not related to the Hatha yoga practices; rather, it is concerned with attaining a steady, comfortable position to be used exclusively for meditation. Some schools of meditation are currently advocating the use of Western-style chairs for meditation, stating that it isn't altogether necessary to sit cross-legged in the typical Indian manner. I don't totally disagree with this position, though I strongly believe there are benefits in sitting cross-legged in either the half-lotus or full-lotus posture. I know of no other position for meditation more stable than this one. Sitting on the floor gives the aspirant a feeling of being rooted to the earth, a sensation that prepares him for deep and powerful experiences. On a chair, this feeling is just not there; you are raised above the ground; your legs being of no supportive value. While sitting on the floor, the back can be held straight, with the chest held up. This provides for a free flow of energy up and down the spine.

All of the aforementioned can be maintained while in a chair; however, some of us tend to slump over, round our shoulders, and tuck in our chins. An additional point to make note of is that sitting in a chair is more conducive to sleep than sitting cross-legged on the floor. And believe me, when first starting meditation, sleep is one of the most difficult things to fight off, especially in the morning. In no way do I wish to mitigate the difficulty of the cross-legged poses, especially in the beginning; for a while, everything will hurt. Your legs will fall asleep, your back and buttocks will hurt, your shoulders will ache, and parts of the body you have never felt before will suddenly cry out for attention. There are Hatha yoga postures that help alleviate these discomforts by stretching out the muscles and making them more flexible.

Sitting. Sit on a soft blanket that has been folded several times; this provides a soft cushion which elevates the buttocks and helps the knees touch the floor. After crossing your legs, push both the chest and the pelvis out; this maintains your balance and displaces some of the pressure from the buttocks onto the knees. It may help, at the start of the practice, to sit with your back against the wall, not using it as a support, but rather as an aid in keeping the back straight. A hint: if your back touches the wall, you know you are slumping and therefore straighten up. However, a ramrod straight back is not our goal. It should be as straight as possible, while maintaining a comfortable, relaxed pose. Stretch your legs occasionally. This will decrease the chances of their falling asleep. Do this only when you have to, working on spreading the times intervals out until you hardly need to stretch at all. Remember, the asanas of the Hatha yoga system are designed to assist in these particular areas. The leg stretches of the forward bending poses, in particular, give the practitioner a flexible body for meditation. Practice sitting cross-legged while you are doing something else, such as reading. It will be less tedious and you will be able to sit for longer periods of time and get quicker results. Also, simply sitting on the floor as much as possible is a good means of preparation.

Attaining the proper posture takes preparation and work, but it is important to perfect it, for without a steady seat, nothing can really be accomplished in meditation. So, to the best of your ability, follow these basic hints. I have seen old and young people, after several months of practice, capable of sitting cross-legged in meditation for a relatively long duration of time, without discomfort. As your legs and back gain in flexibility, you can wean yourself from the aids mentioned here.

Pranayama, relationship to meditation. Pranayama is the fourth limb. The Hatha yoga section has covered some of the aspects of pranayama. For those of you who haven't read that section, I will briefly review some of the principles.

There is a vital force that springs from the self, Atman. This force releases energy, a manifestation of prana. Prana is the foundation, the core of the manifested universe. In other words, the universe we know and perceive springs from, and is connected by, it.

Mind and prana. Prana is related to the mind, and through the mind, to the will; and through the will, to the individual soul; and through the soul, to the supreme being. Mind, will, thought, soul, and supreme being are interconnected, through prana, to the rest of the manifested universe. The interconnections are both horizontal and vertical.

Control of prana. Once you learn to control the waves of the mind, which are manifestations of prana (commonly referred to as thoughts), you are able to control universal prana. Control of prana is pranayama. Why do we want to control it? By controlling prana, we can regulate the mind. With command over the mind, we are able to experience self. That is yoga.

Pranayama and kundalini. Kundalini is a spiritual force that lies at the base of the spine while in its dormant stage. It can be raised by various spiritual disciplines, i.e, violent breathing practices or mantras. In most people, it ascends and descends between the first three chakras. (See below for explanation of chakras.) Only in evolved spiritual beings does it rise higher.

The raising of kundalini through all seven chakras opens the deep realms of the superconscious to the aspirant.

Nadis. The pranic force flows through subtle, invisible nerve tubes called nadis.

The chakras. Several nadis interlace through seven specific areas in the body called chakras. Three important nadis—the Sushumna, the Ida, and the Pingala—run closely along the spine. The Sushumna is within the spinal canal, the Ida originates from the left nostril, and the Pingala from the right. These nadis interlace seven times as they go through the seven chakras. The chakras are located at various parts of the body: the base of the spine, underneath the genitals, below the navel, in the center of the chest, bottommost tip of the neck, between the eyebrows, and at the crown of the head.

Optimal situation. When the breath operates through the Sushumna, the mind becomes steady. If, however, the nadis have impurities in them, the breath cannot pass through this middle nadi, thus causing the mind to become cloudy and unbalanced. The practice of pranayama is useful in purifying the nadis and making the breath flow evenly and calmly.

Pranayama and breath, the control of breath. Breath, the external manifestation of prana, is linked to the more subtle element of prana, the thoughts. The control of breath (a gross prana) leads to power over its more elusive counterparts, the mind and its thoughts.

Pranayama as an aid. Pranayama performs either one of two functions: it moves the mind in an upward direction, or it calms the mind. It is an aid to the full evolution of the self. Pranayama, itself, will not give realization, but in the hands of the sincere aspirant, it can be a very useful tool.

When and where to do pranayama. It is best, since pranayama raises the heat in the system, to practice it in a cool and quiet place, preferably a shaded area. The aspirant should not have eaten for some time prior to commencing the practice. As I've previously indicated, pranayama is helpful in making one's meditation peaceful.

Pranayama exercises. The following pranayama can be viewed as additions to those already mentioned in the Hatha yoga section. The first two pranayamas, bastrikas and suka purvaka, are extensions of kapalabhati and nadi suddhi. (See Hatha yoga section for description of latter two.)

Rousing the mind, bastrikas. Before meditation, it is advisable to do three rounds of bastrikas, which resemble kapalabhati in many ways. The main differences between bastrikas and kapalabhati is that kapalabhati places more force on the exhalation, as well as having a period of breath retention. Like kapalabhati, you sit with the back straight and head erect. The power for forcing the air out the nose comes from the abdomen. The head, neck, and shoulders remain still; only the abdomen moves, puffing up and pushing the air out. Start off slowly, then gradually increase to a round of about twenty to twenty-five breaths. In the beginning, start off with no more than ten. After the last exhalation in the round, take a deep breath and hold it, while tucking your chin into your chest. After a few seconds, slowly raise your chin and exhale through your nose. While you exhale, feel the pranic energy rush up and out the top of your head.

Calming the mind, nadi suddhi and suka purvaka. Suka purvaka is nadi suddhi in conjunction with breath retention and a maintenance of a specific ratio of exhalations to inhalations. Nadi suddhi is performed by first placing the thumb on the right nostril, then exhaling fully out the left side. This is followed by taking a deep breath, closing off the left nostril, and exhaling out the right side in succession. You execute the same procedure in suka purvaka, with only the following variation: the ratio and retention are different. In this practice, you breathe out the left nostril, take a deep breath, then pinch both nostrils closed. After a short interval, open up the right nostril and breathe out. Follow this by taking a deep breath through the right side, then closing off both nostrils again. Hold your breath for a few seconds, then exhale through the left side. The ideal ratio for suka purvaka is 1:4:2; for beginners, a ratio of 1:2:2 may be more comfortable. Translated, this means one count on the inhalation, two for retention, two for exhalation. If, for example, you inhale to a three count, and you are using a 1:2:2 ratio, you would retain your breath for six counts and exhale for six counts. Breathing should not be forced; you should not be gasping for breath every time you inhale. You should strive to progress from the 1:2:2 to the 1:4:2 ratio, working also to increase the count. It is good to hold a mental picture of the breath and its movement in relation to prana. Inhale, the prana travels down to the base of the spine. Exhale, prana rises up and out the top of the head. During retention, focus your attention on the upper four chakras: the heart, the throat, between the eyebrows, and the top of the head.

Meditative pranayama. Deerghaswasam, deep breathing, is a meditative pranayama we've already discussed. Breath goes down to the abdomen, lungs, and chest, successively, and is exhaled in the reverse order: chest, lungs, abdomen. This breathing practice should be done using a 1:2 ratio. One-count inhalation to two-count exhalation. Ujjayi pranayama is another meditative pranayama. Ujjayi, the "hissing breath," is breathing slowly through the nose while keeping the mouth closed. You should feel the air hiss past the epiglottis, right behind the nasal passages. It should sound like soft snoring. This breath should be done in conjunction with deerghaswasam. The third type of meditative pranayama is brahmari, the "humming breath." It is performed with both the lips and eyes closed. First you inhale deeply, keeping the lips closed. You vibrate the upper palate on the exhalation. This breath can also be done with the yoni mudra. In the mudra, you close off the eyes and the ears in order to allow you to focus more directly on the vibration that is produced. You should feel the vibration rise up and fill the entire head. If done properly, the entire system should vibrate. After several rounds of this pranayama, a peaceful meditation can be realized rather quickly and easily.

The cooling breaths, sitali and sitkari. The "cooling breaths" lower the heat in the body system. In doing sitali, curl your tongue and suck air through it. Close your mouth and retain the breath for a few moments, then exhale through the nose. For those unable to curl their tongue in this manner, sitkari can be practiced. Sitkari is very similar; here, however, the tongue is curled behind clenched teeth. Other than the addition of clenching the teeth, the procedure is the same. On a hot day, both breathing techniques can cool the system and bring saliva to a parched mouth.

Pranayama and meditation routine. I've found the following pranayama routine the best to prepare for meditation. First, do three rounds of bastrikas to rouse the mind out of its tamasic aspect. Then do five rounds of suka purvaka. (As you become more advanced, you'll find you can add more rounds.) If you desire, you can then add the ujjayi and brahmari pranayamas. This procedure should prepare you for a good and deep meditation.

Pratyahara, sense control, the fifth limb.

Some background. I remember hearing a story, some years ago, about a group of people who were trying to give up smoking cigarettes. They formed a circle, into the center of which someone threw a pack of cigarettes. The leader of the session looked at the group and asked them, "Who is the master, you or that pack of cigarettes?" A woman quickly responded, "Well, I know who is; it's that little cigarette pack!" Control of the senses has become an issue of high priority, not only for yogis, but for the population at large. In this society, in which so much is made available, the tendency to overindulge is prevalent. That is why it has become important for us to look toward the practice of pratyahara. If people practiced this discipline to begin with, there would probably be no need for the plethora of health clubs and diet plans that exist today. While other nations are starving,

Americans are spending millions of dollars to take off that which they so immoderately put on. But there are other examples too. The man with the "roving eye" and the person who is constantly drawn to shop windows are people inflicted with poor sense control. Our eyes, ears, and tongues are literally leading us down the physical, mental, and moral drain. What can we do? We can't escape from the world by hiding in a cave. We must deal with the world as it is. And looking at what progress has brought us in the last fifty years, there are apt to be objects made that will be even more enticing, tempting us to seek greater pleasure by possessing them. Until ultimately, like material junkies, we are the ones possessed. How can we resolve the conflict of sense control in a world that is actively trying to subvert it? Before we come to any conclusions, or even make any hypotheses, let us first see what pratyahara is.

Pratyahara. This is the practice of withdrawal, or control of the senses, from sense objects. This is not, and should not, be mistaken for an ascetic discipline. Properly practical, this is a means to moderately control the senses. When we talk about controlling or withdrawing the senses, we do not mean retreating from or repressing them. Some yoga students do the latter; it is not the fault of the practice, but rather of the students.

The main aid in sense control is a purified mind. Once the mind is pure, that which is filtered into it by the senses will be perceived correctly. The individual will then know whether something is or is not good for the body and mind, whether it will bring pain or peace. The all-important element of attachment is again placed foremost before the mind. The mind must be able to discern whether the object perceived by the senses is good for the body and itself. It will know that if something is pleasurable, its tendency will be to attach to it. But a great pain could result from this attachment, the pain of separation, if for some reason the object of pleasure was taken away. That is why the mind as a pure receptacle for the sense impressions is so important in pratyahara. Control and leadership cannot come from a clouded mind. And if the individual is oriented toward self, he will know that sense objects are merely transitory pleasures.

Benefits. The benefits of pratyahara are great. The mind becomes peaceful and receptive to deep concentration. Focus can be maintained, no matter what the task or the surrounding of the practitioner is. I've seen this discipline in my own teacher; in the midst of a crowd of people, he is able to converse with not only one person, but two or three, on as many subjects. The person who practices pratyahara is like a tortoise; he carries his shell with him, able at any time to draw his limbs and senses from stimulants.

Samyam, the three final rungs.

Dharana, concentration. Dharana is fixing the mind on one point, object, or idea and holding it there. The path to successful meditation starts with dharana. For, in essence, to meditate is to practice dharana successfully. The difficulty in meditation is maintaining the mind on one point. The mind wanders, thus the constant task of the meditator is to bring it back to the point of concentration. This very act of bringing the mind back to a single point helps increase the power of focus. Our lives are full of experiences of dharana. Reading is such an example. In the beginning, your mind may be distracted by the physical surroundings; but after several attempts at bringing the mind back to focus, you become so absorbed in what is on the page that even breathing slows down. You lose awareness of the outside world and become wholly engrossed in the book. Pratyahara, dharana, dhyana, and samadhi are no different from engrossed reading. In pratyahara, we withdraw our senses from the outside world. In dharana, we focus on one point. In dhyana, our concentration is uninterrupted and engrossed, and in samadhi, we are wholly submerged and absorbed into the point of concentration. Once a point of concentration is chosen, spiritual practice naturally moves ahead with a great deal of fervor. We can choose an external object for concentration, like a picture of a teacher or deity, a candle flame, or the central spot of a mandalic design; or we can focus on an internal point, such as a mantra, breath, a chakra, or an inner ideal. The most important criteria to use in selecting a point of concentration is that the "object" be pleasing and spiritually significant to the mind. In the beginning, the mind will rebel against the practice; it will work to block and interfere with the spiritual progress. This is because the mind will be losing control, as the self slowly begins to affect control over it. The mind will fight this loss of power. No individual, group, or country ever gives up power willingly, and neither does the mind. Some aspirants complain of ill health, disturbing nightmares, severe doubts. These are all attempts by the mind to subvert the spiritual practice. Grooves have to be cut into the mind by the initial practice of concentration; this in itself takes several months of steady practice. There is no need to be terribly concerned if the mind continues to "run away" repeatedly, especially in the beginning. The practice takes considerable time to become fully established.

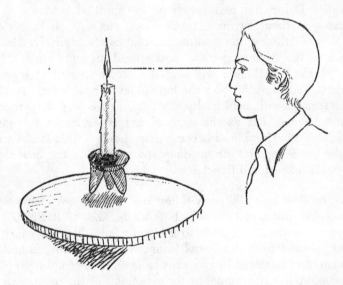

Tradak. Another means of increasing the power of concentration is by practicing tradak. One performs tradak by gazing at a candle placed at eye level. Use a candle that gives a steady flame; place it in an area where the air is still. Look at the flame with eyes wide open for thirty to sixty seconds, or until your eyes begin to tear. With eyes closed, visualize the flame between your eyebrows. Hold the image for as long as possible. Tradak can also be done using a picture, though this may take a more advanced power of concentration.

Further hints. There is no doubt that real advancement in raja yoga cannot occur without serious training of the afore-mentioned procedures of the moral and ethical practices. If the impurities are not removed first, during these steps, they tend to become magnified during the practice of concentration. Imagine, for example, an individual who has not fully worked out his tendency toward greed and selfishness but has nevertheless increased his ability to concentrate. The self he will be magnifying through his concentrative powers will be a self clouded with impurities. Delusion, a real danger to true spiritual evolvement, increases. Without having a teacher beforehand, who knows the pitfalls of delusion, the spiritual aspirant can fall terribly. Also, if some of the beginning moral and ethical precepts are not followed, the practitioner will find it difficult to perfect concentration. For no matter how the individual tries to focus, thoughts and feelings will continually crop up, subverting the process. Some believe that as the aspirant comes closer to the goal, difficulties and problems become more intense. This is not true. If the beginning and intermediary steps are done, the final steps virtually take care of themselves.

Dhyana and samadhi, meditation and absorption. Dhyana is prolonged concentration, which flows in and of itself. Often, dhyana has been compared to a viscous fluid, like oil, which is being poured from one vessel to another in a steady, unbroken stream. As I've stated before, dhyana is a result of uninterrupted concentration. Ajapa japa, or the repetition of the mantra without conscious volition, is a form of dhyana. When dhyana occurs, breath becomes very slow, verging on stopping altogether. Thoughts subside. A transcendent peace descends upon all understanding. The meditative object, which has been the subject of prolonged, continued focus, shines forth in its real nature during this state of peace. Suddenly, the mantra takes on a unique significance never before seen. The breath, the candle flame are understood in a new light, a much deeper and meaningful way. It is not an understanding that comes from a single surface analysis; rather, it draws from within. Meditation has been described as a "peak experience." It is that, and more. Peak experiences usually do not last for any great length of time. Depending on one's ability to concentrate during meditation, a peak experience may be from one to ten minutes in duration. There have even been cases in which great spiritual teachers have stayed in meditation for considerably longer periods. Meditation, once entered, is transforming to both the mind and body. Having perfected the ability to meditate, the student is ready for samadhi: absorption. Absorption comes about from prolonged meditation. It is where thoughts subside completely, and the mind achieves or realizes a feeling of oneness with the meditation object. In other words, samadhi is an extension of the meditative act. There are, however, a few lower forms of samadhi, in which the mind still perceives the object of meditation with an awareness of its name, quality, and function. There is absorption, but it is still tinged with a consciousness of its physical properties and manifestation. Only in the highest samadhi, Nirvakalpa or seedless samadhi, is there purified, undiluted, undifferentiated awareness. At this level, there is neither object nor subject, just an unending awareness. This experience, which is the pinnacle of most spiritual practices, has been poetically described as oceanic in depth and brighter than a thousand suns. The name is Sanskrit for those who have received this intense experience is "jivanmukta," or liberated living beings. Their karma (past impressions) are wiped out, freeing them from the realms of birth and death. (We will discuss this in greater depth in the Karma yoga section.) The knowledge received from entering absorption, is close to impossible to communicate. It can neither be gotten from a book nor a spiritual study. Samadhi is the experience most yoga practitioners strive to attain. But it only can be arrived at after much hard work. Swami Sivananda put it succinctly, "To meditate is easy, but to prepare for meditation is hard." What kind of yogi one is depends greatly on how well he has prepared himself. Samadhi is a lifelong commitment; anyone who strives for it by putting little or no work into the endeavor is merely fooling himself. It is a life sentence, so to speak. It may even be considered a multiple life sentence, because the striving for deep understanding is something that goes beyond just one life. But samadhi is not the end of the yoga practice. Samadhi is important for how it will be used, as well as its intrinsic value. It is said, the only way an individual can come back, after receiving a deep samadhilike experience, is by dedicating him or herself completely to humanity. Thus, samadhi is at once one of the greatest experiences of self, which is wholly selfish, and at the same time one of the greatest experiences of humanity, the fullest expression of selflessness.

Occurrences of samadhi are not the complete providence of Indian holy men. There have been many Westerners who have experienced samadhi. Sivananda pointed out that Benjamin Franklin was such a person. Andrew Greely, in a recent Sunday New York *Times Magazine,* wrote that America is fastly becoming a nation of mystics, many of whom have experienced great "oceanic" spiritual occurrences. How, you may ask, can people experience such happenings without ever practicing yoga? Perhaps they never practiced formal yoga, but that does not negate the possibility of its principles from being followed in other ways. Yoga is not wholly a unique practice; aspects of it can be found in people's daily lives around the world. One has only to look at the compassionate neighbor, or a contemplative friend who knows little about formal spirituality, to realize that spirit evolves in truly mysterious ways. We should not be so vain as to think that none can enter Him except through yoga.

chapter four — Head Work, Hide and Seek

There is a nice, illustrative story dealing with why man is in the position he is, in relation to God, and what a jnana yogi must do to find God. As the story goes, there were some angels, relatively high up on the organizational ladder, who were trying to decide where to hide God, now that the earth had been created. They knew that some curious creatures called human beings existed on earth. And having studied their behavior, the angels were sure the creatures would quickly destroy God out of curiosity and ignorance. So they wanted to hide God in such a place where man would never find Him.

"Why don't we put God down under the sea?" suggested the first angel. "No, that's no good," emphatically stated the second angel. "Knowing man, he'll devise a way to get down there." The first angel, undaunted, made another suggestion, "What about in the sky, way up, higher than the moon?" "No," mused the second one dejectedly, "these human beings are very inventive and ingenious; they'll probably find some means to get up into the high sky." The first angel, now showing signs of stress, blurted out,

"There doesn't seem to be any place we can put Him, neither the depths of the sea nor the heights of the sky seem to be out of the realm of man. Where can we put God?" The third angel, having listened quietly and closely to the above discussion, announced that he knew where to put God. "Where?" queried the others. "It's really quite simple. Put God *inside* of man. He will never look there. These humans are always looking outside for everything; outside for solutions to their problems, outside for satisfaction of their desires. Man will never find God inside himself."

Jnana yoga is a means by which we can go within, sever the unreal from the real, and find God. Jnana yoga is the path of self-analysis. The principle tool of the jnana yogi is his intellect; he uses it like a knife, cutting away the non-reality from the unchanging, absolute reality. First, prior to discussing Jnana yoga, let us define the terms "real" and "unreal."

What is real?   A disciple once asked the great teacher, Shankaracharya, what the opposite of dualism was. He answered, "It is not two." He specifically didn't say it was one, for "one" still presents you with a dualistic conception, yourself and the "one." Reality is non-dual. It is beyond the conception of you and me, this and that, black and white. It is beyond all the pairs of opposites that link the visible, physical, and mental world. So if we ask ourselves, "What is reality?", we can simply respond, in the most non-dualistic manner, "That which is real is not unreal." It is, however, difficult to fathom, with our dualistically constructed mind, the reality that stretches beyond it. Simply put, that which is real is permanent; that which changes is unreal. All men strive for a permanent base of understanding. Living in a world of constant change, man, throughout the ages, has searched for a permanence, an underlying truth in his life. The quest for happiness is really a quest for the changeless. Even more than happiness, man seeks to understand that which is beyond his own changing condition, his death. And the search for life after death, too, is a search for the changeless. First, before we know the real, we must transcend the unreal. And this cannot be done until false ideas such as false individualism, identification, and attachment are given up. These ideas foster ignorance, which binds and holds the aspirant to the unreal world. Through self-analysis, the aspirant utilizes his mind and especially his intellect, to sever the mind from those false ideas. In essence, the mind in all its multiplicity, works on itself. It is important to stress here that the mind never does, nor can it, conceptualize reality. However, if it is properly trained, it can "lend a hand" and lead the individual to reality. The first step to work on in the process of self-analysis is conceptualizing the idea of reality. Using the mind, the aspirant sets up and categorizes the dualistic structure of "real" and "unreal." As a conceptualization, reality at this point is just as unreal as non-reality.

Mind-conceptualized reality.

Matter. We'll begin with our physical world, that which our five senses can perceive. Our physical universe is composed of an astronomical number of minute particles of matter. This is a truth we accept, not simply because scientists tell us so, but because with our own senses, we hear, see, touch, and smell the elements of the universe come together, dissolve, and metamorphose. Many forms of matter will melt when heated. There is such matter that will decay and decompose (or in other words, chemically react with other matter or elements) with age. Some will alter shape by the mere exposure to air (which is itself, after all, a composite of elements). Thus, since matter has the property of being in a state of constant change, it does not fit our definition of reality. Energy, too, must be rejected, since it, more than the matter it composes, takes on new forms constantly. When water freezes and becomes ice, both the molecular structure and the amount of energy in the hydrogen and oxygen molecule change.

Astral body. With the rejection of matter as reality, let us focus our attention on the bright body which supposedly exists, even after the physical body is gone. It was postulated a long time ago that this astral body was reality, the fountainhead of the divine spirit of man. Later on, philosophers discarded this belief because if, in fact, the astral body was a form, it was impermanent by its very nature. And like the physical body, the astral body needed an underlying reality to either manipulate it, or have it manifested. Under close analysis, the astral body was discovered to be the receptacle of the mind and thus, as a physical entity, changeable.

Atman. Looking past the astral body, beyond the mind, yogis discovered something that was infinite. It was a spirit shared by all men and all things. This reality existed both within and beyond the mind. But as long as men lived solely within the mind, they would be bound, because the mind changed "infinite" into "finite" by the nature of its structure, which exists in the confines of a space-time continuum. However, this reality, the atman, is a changeless state in which everything hangs in perfect precision. Even though outer forms of objects, elements, and people change, their inner nature is essentially the same in all. It is in this perfect precision that all elements exist in reality. This great force that creates, binds, and destroys manipulates the universe through its slow evolution. All the changes of the universe are the manifestations of this one single force. Only in the mind are we separate, autonomous entities; in reality, we are all one and interconnected. The individual perception of spirit is Atman; the unmanifested spirit is Brahman.

What is unreal? In Jnana yoga we are primarily concerned with what is unreal, rather than real. The reasoning for this goes as follows: we cannot conceptualize reality, we can conceptualize non-reality. Since our task is to sever ourselves from the latter, it is best we become fully cognizant of all its manifestations. With that understanding, we will know what must be wiped out, to enable us to realize and experience the underlying reality. There are three main aspects of unreality: false individualism, false identification, and false attachment. These three categories fall under the general classification of maya. We will now discuss and look closer at the many parts which comprise maya.

Individualism. Individualism is an attribute keenly developed in Western society. To be a "rugged individualist" is, among other things, to feel a kinship to those that founded this country. Today, people go to encounters, marathons, and therapies to strengthen their individuality. Why do so many people search so desperately for their own individualism and are so fearful of losing it, say, in a relationship, a commitment, or a spiritual practice? What does this word individuality mean, and why is it considered unreal?

Body individuality. Many people identify their bodies with their individuality. Often we base our separateness on our body changes as we get older. There are specific rites of passage which ceremonialize the different stages the body goes through in the aging process. Each age has its mores, behavior patterns, and place in the community hierarchy. If I am older, I am a parent, I am a grandparent, I am an elder statesman; I deserve respect. If I am younger, I am beautiful, I am active, I am rebellious; I want change. Whether I am old or young, I want to be with individuals like myself. Young people don't want to be with old people; old people are intolerant of the young. Here then is individualism based on age. The body also presents itself in color and shape; additional aspects for individualism to "hang its hat on." Fat people feel insecure in comparison to thin people; blacks are discriminated against by whites. We separate ourselves into camps, based on our individual physical attributes. We think of ourselves as separate, and because we identify with our bodies, we are separate.

Habits. There are many among us who fervently believe that our particular habits are what make us different and uniquely ourselves. I am an individual because of what I do. But is it the dirt, the long hair, the drugs, and the disengaged attitude that make a street person? What if you clean one up; will that person lose his or her individuality along with the dirt? And how many of us are really individuals if we stick closely to those friends who have habits like ourselves?

Memory. Is individuality a function of memory? If I became amnesiac, would I lose my individuality? Memories are constantly being altered by time; so how can anyone pin his individuality on such a high variable?

People tend to see individuality on their own terms. They are frightened of large changes (the small everyday alterations they perceive as no change) and unknown quantities. There is a feeling of safety in holding and maintaining a known, narrow conception of individuality; the parameters are fixed, the risks are minimized. False individuality is a crisis in courage and vision.

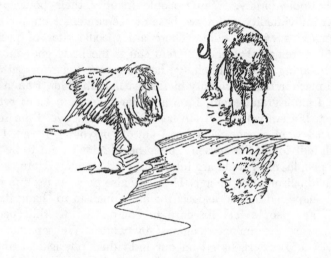

Identification. The story about the lion who was raised by sheep is apropos to a discussion of this topic. A young lion's mother was shot and killed by a hunter, and the orphaned cub, in its wanderings, found its way to some nearby grazing sheep. One of the ewes in the flock adopted the cub and took care of it as one of its own. The lion, being young and impressionable, soon began to assume a sheeplike behavior: it bleated and walked like a sheep and played gently with the lambs. Well, as the story goes, one day when it was a grown and mature lion, it happened into the forest where it came upon another lion. It started to run away in fear that the other lion would attack and eat it. "What are you doing?" questioned the forest lion in some puzzlement at his behavior. "Why are you running away?" The sheeplike lion looked at him incredulously. "Obviously because you are a lion and you will eat me." "What do you mean?" said the other. "We're both lions aren't we? Why would I want to eat you?" "I'm not a lion," our sheeplike friend protested. "I'm a sheep." "You are not," said the other somewhat humored by this statement. "You're a lion, just as I am. Come over here and I'll prove it to you." He took him to a nearby pond. And what he beheld in the reflection of the still water was two lions staring up at him. And in recognition, he roared out, "I AM A LION!" This little parable illustrates exactly what occurs in false identification. We choose to identify with something that is less than our full totality of being. We are indeed fuller and more complete than how we identify ourselves. There are two principle forms false identification takes, the body and the mind.

Body identification. To some extent, we all identify with our bodies. Most of us actually believe we are our bodies. For instance, someone asks, "Who are you?" You respond, "I am so-and-so, and I am such an age." Essentially, you are giving your body's name and age. If, however, we identify ourselves with our spirit, atman, we have no birthday, and we have no name. This does not deny that, to a large extent, we live in the world of bodies. When a fellow body dies a physical death, we grieve; when a fellow body is born into our world, we rejoice. My teacher often has commented on this process, calling it backward and contrary to the actual rewards and punishments of the two events. He questions it thusly, "Why do we feel such grieving when someone leaves? This is insanity. This world is a madhouse." He says, "If we could see the view from the other side, after death, the person leaving the world would probably be happy. And if we could place ourselves into the head of a newborn infant, we would see that the child is crying at being placed in this insane-asylumlike world. We are happy at its arrival because it is another individual sharing the insanity with us. When someone leaves, we grieve because he has escaped from the madhouse, abandoning us to stick it out without him."

Some people glorify their identification with their bodies by excessive preoccupation with their physical mien. These individuals sometimes go through considerable emotional changes over their body as it ages. This is one of the reasons why one has to take care in the practice of Hatha yoga, for as one develops an awareness of body, there is a tendency to become preoccupied with the look and shape of it. Perfection in the body is not perfection in the soul. It is relatively easy to attain perfection in the body; it is a much harder task to realize it in the spirit.

Mind: self-concept and ideology.

Self-concept. How a person thinks of himself is determined by his past and his perceptions of the experiences that comprise it. Perceptions are affected by one's temperament, which, in turn, are affected by karma—the individual's past actions. Discussion of karma will follow in the next chapter. Self-concept can trap you in a vicious cycle; thoughts produce actions, actions are analyzed by perceptual powers colored by a temperament that has been affected by previous actions. For example, if a person has a poor self-concept, his actions will be performed under a strong expectation of failure. When one case after another of failure occurs, they gather and form into a temperament of failure; thus you have the classical "hard-luck case." With that temperament and built-up perception, the person perceives himself and his actions as failures. This, in turn, falls back onto the self-concept, which again repeats the cycle.

What this means. It is difficult to break through the self-concept, whether it is a healthy or a sick one. To perform this difficult task, the individual must first deal with his mind. Working with the mind means understanding its limitations (which in essence are your own), accepting and not taking them too seriously. A good self-concept is important (it is, after all, better than having a poor one), but identifying with a healthy self-concept is just as bad as identifying with a sick one. Wear your self-concept lightly, for it is only a conception, and whatever is conceived is changeable. Contemporary psychoanalysis and therapy function, among other things, in providing the individual with a healthy self-concept. Therapy provides tools for the individual to use in coping with reality. Being able to successfully deal with reality consequently affects and alters the self-concept. However, in most contemporary psychology, no thought is given to transcending the self-concept.

Ideology. Ideology is incorporated in the self-concept. It can take many forms; political, religious, philosophical, psychological. Here, we of course are referring to the spiritual form. Ideology can help us explain our relationship to the world, though we should be wary of identifying too closely with it. In the beginning, however, it may be necessary to internalize the message of the ideology, to become a wholehearted adherent of its precepts. In some individuals, a prolonged exposure to an ideology produces a deep attachment to it; this attachment may lead to its internalization as the self-concept. An ideology should be looked at as a tool, a means to an end, not the end in itself. Ideologies are ways of explaining different aspects of the world. Inclusively, they are not reality itself, but they do point a way to a particular reality. Yoga is nothing more than an ideology. Many people heavily identify with its ideology. This, of course, is not advisable. In the beginning, one may become very involved with yoga trying to understand the practices and to internalize them; you should never forget that to be a yogi, you must be yourself. And to be yourself, completely, is to be a yogi. Perceiving the world through yoga-colored "glasses" is just as unreal as to perceive it through any other highly ideologically colored "glasses." My teacher metaphorically refers to yoga as a mind cleanser. But, he also reminds us, soap itself is a kind of dirt, and in the end, it too must be rinsed away.

Attachment. Once Indra, a Hindu deity-king, planned to exhibit his powers to the hierarchy of deities. He announced that he wanted to know what it would be like to be a pig, and the only way to know such a thing would be to become one. All the deities pleaded with him not to do this. But he disregarded their entreaties, assuring them that he would be able to remember his identity and not become heavily attached in being and understanding the pig. So Indra took birth as a pig. He lived very contentedly in the pigpen in a farmer's barnyard. After some time, the farmer placed a young female pig in with him. They became friendly and raised a family. Now he was even more happy than he had been when alone. Every day he wallowed in the mud, enjoying its coolness. He totally loved the life of a pig. Then one day, the farmer came along, took the young piglets and slit their throats; and Indra became terribly sad and grief-stricken. The

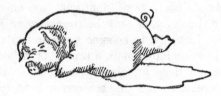

next day the farmer came back, took the wife away and slit her throat too. Now Indra was beside himself with grief. He was in such a state of bereavement that the deities decided he was too involved in his pig experiment; so, as he was grieving, they came down and cut his pig body. When Indra reappeared as himself, he realized in an instant how deep and all-consuming his attachment had been.

Attachment is often difficult to comprehend. Society often encourages attachment, i.e., to family, wealth, and position. It exists in, and works through, the mind. Many people feel that if they give away everything, they will no longer be attached. But the mind has its own attachments. You can give away everything and remain tied not to "things" but to the very act of non-attachment. This kind of attachment is extremely hard to extricate, since it is based on nothing in the physical world. Material objects can be taken away, but an attachment that exists solely in the mind is often carefully protected by internal defense mechanisms.

Once there were two monks living in a secluded part of the forest. One was an ascetic who lived a very rigorous-type existence in a cave and whose only possession was a solitary water pot, used for drinking and washing his hands. The other monk also lived in a cave, but his cave was really quite comfortable, with all the modern conveniences—wall-to-wall carpets, TV, air conditioner. This monk also had his family come up quite frequently to visit him. The ascetic monk used to make fun of the worldly monk by kidding him about his material attachments. One day, the two were sitting in the worldly monk's cave, discussing spiritual matters, when the ascetic monk launched into an elaborate description about the beauty and spirituality of Rishikesh, a town many hundreds of miles away, in the foothills of the Himalayas. In the middle of this description, the worldly monk jumped up and said, "Let's go right now." And he grabbed his shawl and went rushing out through the door. The other monk was completely surprised by the other's actions, but he followed nonetheless. They hadn't walked very far when the ascetic monk stopped suddenly. "Oh my goodness, I must go back to my cave," he cried. "Why?" said the other. "I forgot my water pot; I never go out without it," he replied. The worldly monk turned around and smiled. "After all your kidding about my worldly attachments, you seem to be more attached to that solitary pot than I to all my possessions."

Attachment begins when the individual can no longer face the pain of existence. As infants, we are biologically and psychically attached to our mothers. Unless we are, we will perish or suffer significant psychological damage. There have been several studies done on the effects of maternal deprivation on infants. It has been found that infants need maternal attachment. But, because of this early life need, we set up a modality of attachment which we continue to apply to our adult years. For, whenever we face that pain, the pain of first entering this world, we look for attachments to alleviate it. Attachments vary; there are positive, real ones, and there are negative, false ones. Attachments which lead toward a disinterested, but involved, life are best. Sivananda said, "Detach the mind from the world and attach it to the

Lord." This kind of attachment is pure and liberating. False attachments, however, are delusionary; they give you a sense of freedom without granting you the freedom itself. They may give you more space to buy off imminent pain, but in the end, the pain from the "disattaching" process causes a greater hurt than the camouflaged pain. Often people with monetary wealth feel they can achieve independence with it. They claim to feel free and unattached. But are they really? Say someone owns a Lincoln Continental, a home in the country, and a duplex in the city. Supposedly he has no worries and is secure in the freedom his wealth buys him. I would imagine that he would suddenly feel extremely attached if the Lincoln was stolen or if the summer house was set ablaze by arson. Such people often claim that they are free but are really slaves to "their" material objects. They say that their interest for these "toys" wears off quickly, and they must go out to find something else that is more exciting. Haven't they truly put themselves in bondage? By these statements I don't mean to imply that I am against having material objects or, for that matter, family relationships. Rather, one should strive to extinguish the feeling of ownership too often inherent in these relationships. Instead of "ownership," cultivate the feeling of caretakership—a temporary management in which you know full-well that the objects and the people neither belong nor are obligated to you and, in all likelihood, will someday leave you. After all, we all know, at least intellectually, that family members grow up, age, and pass on, just as material objects get old, decay, and pass on. It is common for people who become attached to objects to seek substitutes for those "possessions" that have been taken away or removed from their sphere of influence. If substitutes are unavailable, and the number of attachments continue to diminish, the importance of those left can rise proportionately. Remember the monk and the water pot? The kind of attachment he exhibited is difficult to discover and even more difficult to irradicate. My teacher frequently recommends a little test to people who wish to know how many attachments they have. First, they should ask themselves, "Who am I?" A sample response may be: father, son, brother, fireman, community leader; all the roles played at that given moment in the person's life. Swamiji suggests that the larger and more extensive the list, the further the person is from understanding himself. Equipped with this additional knowledge, the aspirant can apply the jnana yogi's principal tool for severing attachment: neti-neti. Neti is Sanskrit for "not this." When a person is confronted with whom he thinks he is, he says, "Not this." He says, "Not this," to all things and to all conceptions, until he has successfully severed himself from all the formalized conceptions and broken through the barrier to the real inner being.

Maya. As you see, the concepts of individualism, false identification, and false attachment overlap one another. An individual attached to his individualism usually identifies himself with a concept or an ideology, thus re-enforcing his individualism. Any attachment or identification with a concept or an ideology separates rather than unites. For example, novice yoga students sometimes set themselves apart from non-yoga people. They feel they have special knowledge and are therefore special themselves. They identify with this particular self-concept and the ideology of yoga. Consequently, these new aspirants become very attached to the practice and the "specialness" surrounding it. This behavior is contrary to spiritual progress. Collectively, this state of delusion is called maya. Maya is more than a state of delusion; it is an all-encompassing web that imprisons man. It is a feeling of doomed certainty "that time and tide will take all men"; a feeling of inexorable entrapment that may force man to seek pleasure and abandonment in an attempt to abate the feeling. Maya exists deep in the nihilistic attitude of "the world means nothing." Drug addicts, alcoholics, bums, drifters, even some neurotic obese people are all mayic casualties. These people have got trapped and have subsequently entrapped themselves further. But in the midst of this entrapment, in the heart of every man, there exists a feeling of there being more to life. A small voice within cries out, "There must be something beyond this web. There must be a way of getting beyond this feeling that all life is doomed." Here, genuine spiritual search begins. Dissatisfaction must well up in the individual, and he must cry out in desperation and call a halt to his life of sensual enjoyments and cyclical highs and lows. Once the individual hears this voice, *his* voice, and acknowledges it, the road to freedom out of maya becomes visible. In conjunction with this heightened awareness comes a complete understanding of maya. And what maya is, is not all delusionary. Rather, it is a power that forces you to look inward and forces you out of the complacency of your existence, out of your own trap. Once you see maya as the great force of liberation, you have discovered the essence of life's power and plan. Maya, in all its beauty and hideous force, is advancing every sentient being toward liberation. The saint and the sinner, the businessman and the bum, the killed and the killer are all moved by maya's hand, inexorably toward realization. For maya brings an ultimate understanding of freedom as the birthright of all beings; and like automobiles on a huge conveyor belt, we are moving toward completion, whether we like it or not. All of us have experienced tragedy and pain, all have searched for happiness, all have moved from one thing to another, vainly searching, failing, and re-searching. In this light, there is no difference between a bad and a good person. They are both searching for a way out. Perhaps bad stumbles more than good, makes more mistakes; but the difference is a matter of degree and not of kind. At some point, the searcher assumes that God is out there, that there is, indeed, freedom beyond this illusionary world, a freedom beyond nature. Only, however, when man turns within does he see God himself; that realization brings his search and quest to an end. As Swami Vivekananda states, "The God of heaven becomes the God in nature, and the God in nature becomes the God who is nature. And the God who is nature becomes the God within the temple of the body. And the God dwelling in the temple becomes the temple itself, the soul in man." This freedom is with us, within our own hearts. Once freedom is realized and gained, maya no longer has a manipulative power. You can see maya as beautiful, as God's plaything for the evolution of man's spiritual consciousness. Without maya, man would not know his true nature; he would not know his true nature is the very self he is seeking.

chapter five — Selfless Work, the Secret Service

What is Karma yoga? It is the path of selfless action. The essence of Karma yoga is exemplified in the lives of such people as Gandhi, Martin Luther King, Jr., Mother Cabrini, and Sister Kenny, to name a few. What is so unique about their lives which made them capable of transforming so many others?

The essence. Karma yoga is, at its core, surrender and dedication. To become fully selfless and do the divine will, the aspirant surrenders his individuality and personal attachments. With no thought to personal demands, he dedicates himself to a designated task. Coupled with renunciation and dedication is a surrendering of all worldly rewards and/or expectations. Why should people do this? What does it matter if one is attached, or if one wants the fruits of one's labor in the form of money or praise? My teacher draws a pertinent analogy; "If I could talk to an apple tree, I would ask the tree whether it ever eats its own apples. The tree, if it could, would reply, 'No, I just produce apples; that is my job, my duty in this world. I am not like man; only man eats the fruits of his labor.'" The universe, the macrocosm of the apple tree is, at its essence, a constant and beneficent giver that asks for and receives no rewards. All nature conveys this message: the apple tree, the flowers, the sun, all give selflessly of themselves. A flower perfumes the air with its beautiful scent, the sun gives forth rays of warmth and light, and because they give so generously, their needs are filled. Only man is concerned with the returns of his actions. Only man says, "I have to think of number one."

Once there was a man who sat beneath a tree; he laughed hysterically all daylong. The people of his village thought him crazy and left him, more or less, alone. One day, however, a man from a neighboring village, observing this curious behavior, asked the man why he laughed so much. The man looked up and responded cheerfully, "I'm glad you asked me that. You know why I laugh so much? Because I got the best of God." "What are you talking about?" the man asked, incredulous at this statement. The elated man explained, "I made this deal with God; I told God I would give him everything I had; and you know, I don't have very much, just a little house there, and little else. Well, I knew if I gave everything I had to God, God would give everything He had to me. Now I ask you, who got the best end of the deal?" This little story about renunciation shows giving is its own reward; because in giving, one lives in harmony with the rest of the universe, and that is the greatest gift of all. For when you give, you are taken care of by the divine force. Isn't that what Lord Jesus says about the little birds who never worry about food, for God provides them with their necessities? And He will provide you with yours. As long as you give according to the plan, you will get according to the plan.

The ignorance. Because of man's blind and self-indulgent nature, he repeatedly lives in disharmony, both with himself and the universe. Man, in his ignorance, believes he is the doer, the initiator, the one who can maintain things, or destroy them. Man looks at his great technological advances, his cities, and the countries he has built and feels a sense of power and pride in his accomplishments. Man believes he has tamed and even conquered nature. He proudly lords over all his "creations" and says,

"This is all mine." But as he proudly stands over his conquered kingdom, he notices, upon looking closely, that his kingdom is, after all, not his own. He becomes aware that there is no place in his world where the natural forces are not working. His great cities crumble, and his great countries and technologies are powerless in the face of repeated natural phenomena. For man still has not solved the problems of famine, floods, and other natural acts. No one knows yet how to halt the movement of a tornado, nor stop the flow of a volcano. Man somehow fails to relate and recognize the power of this mighty force, even as he prays in church: "Thy will be done on earth, as it is in heaven." Man, locked in his ignorance, constantly faces this superior force, yet still manages to delude himself. Agreed, it is sad, and poignantly tragic, for a family to lose a young child. But how much more tragic it is when the family feels it owns the child and that it was taken away unjustly. Why do people feel the act was unjust? Because they believe they gave life to the child. They raised and nourished it, and therefore they, and only they, should have the final say as to whether the child lives or dies. Unconsciously, people believe, and maintain, this premise. But did the family actually give the child life? It is said that God giveth and God taketh away. If we accept the fact God gives, then it is His right to take away. The fetus is a receptacle for God's giving of life. Often, after a tragic event, in an attempt to "replace the pieces," we square our shoulders and philosophically say, "Life moves on." And isn't that what happens when we bury, in the name of the child, its body? Doesn't its life move on? It is through ignorance that we believe life starts at birth and ends at death; and that we possess the controls governing our lives and our actions. The analogy is made between human destiny and a luxury liner on a cruise. The ship is headed from New York to Gibraltar, but we, the passenger, think that we are doing the moving. We walk along the deck, and go up and down, but our movement will not get the ship to Gibraltar one day sooner or later. And so it is with our lives; we make this choice and that, thinking that it will greatly affect our destiny. But will it? It is like so much "deck walking." Our destiny is on the high seas, and it is steaming into port at its own rate. All that we can do is to stop walking and become aware of the boat's movement.

What is karma? Karma can be split up into three types:

Sanchita karma: The sum total of our actions.

Parabdha karma: The inevitable karma, that action which must be worked out in this lifetime.

Kriyaman karma: That karma which is in the process of being made, actions yet incomplete.

Karma is cyclical. It begins with kriyaman karma, whose actions directly affect parabdha karma. This adds karma to the sum total—the sanchita karma—thus completing and starting the round again. Karma is circular and never-ending. Every time you act, you produce a reaction, thus triggering another action that sets off a reaction, ad infinitum. The entire universe is bound by the laws of karma.

The laws of causation.

The laws of causation are another way of saying the laws of karma. Everything is governed by these laws; all feelings, thoughts, and physiological functions. All of the scientific disciplines and principles pay homage to these laws. Inhalation-exhalation, oxygen changed to carbon dioxide, carbon dioxide changed back to oxygen; all ecology is based on the intricate interdependence of the elements of nature. We cannot make changes in one area of nature without affecting another. The laws of causation affect all areas of nature, including the mind. Everything that is changeable falls under the influence of the laws of causation. It comprises four principal laws: (1) law of action, (2) law of compensation, (3) law of retribution, (4) law of resistance.

(1) The law of action. For every action, there is an equal and just reaction. The laws of physics are particularly exempletive here. One object strikes a static object; it moves with measurable results. Drop a rubber ball to the floor; it bounces up. This law also holds true in the area of interpersonal relations. If you are kind to people, they are kind to you; if you are not, they will reciprocate that behavior. An angry action will produce an angry reaction; for example, in the ecology of mind, angry thoughts harvest an angry personality and vice versa. The emotional vibrations of anger or peace affect the mind, and the results remain to form the sum effect—the sanchita karma. That is why we meditate and do mantra repetition. We try to create peace in the personality, which causes a reaction of peacefulness in the mind. This peacefulness, not to be confused with the peace of realization, is tranquillity; the forerunner of transcendent peace.

(2) The law of compensation. There is balance in the law of nature. This balance is maintained through the law of compensation. Fuel burns and is destroyed; we derive heat and cook our food by it. The mosquito bites us, but he in turn is nourishment for the birds and the fish. In other words, if something happens, it has a compensating effect somewhere else, which maintains the whole system in a state of balance. Sometimes it is difficult to see compensation when things go "wrong," but it is there; we need only look to see it. For years, woodland firefighters thought all fires were harmful to the forests. Years of propaganda and Smokey the Bear reinforced this idea in the minds of the public. Forest rangers and planners now realize this kind of thinking is not necessarily valid. In fact, they now set controlled forest fires to clear the heavy growth of underbrush. Fires are nature's way of cleaning out the garbage of the forests. Man is no different from any other part of nature's world. You may ask, for example, "Why do terrible things happen to me? After all, I lead a good, virtuous life." It is because the law of compensation is at work, and by looking holistically into your life, the full scope of the law will become evident. Always keep in mind no matter what occurs, it is all for the better; it is part of His divine plan. The story of the two brothers depicts this inherent sense of balance in nature. One day, while the men were walking in the forest, one brother caught his arm on a thorn, producing a rather painful wound. The other brother, looking at the blood, laughingly told him, "You know, it is all for good." This statement angered the first brother, and in his rage, he pushed his brother into a well, saying, "You know, if everything is for the good, figure this one out." Laughing, he walked away. Farther down the road, he was captured by a band of cannibals who promptly prepared him for their evening's supper. They were a peculiar tribe, though; they maintained very high standards for their food—no flaws, no discolorations, no bruises. After carefully examining their captive, they discovered the cut on his arm and, disappointed, they quickly released him. Gleefully, the freed man ran back to his brother, who was still in the well. Helping his brother out, he said, "You know, you were right; it really was all for good." "Well, I told you so," said the second. "But," the first one questioned, "if everything is for good, what was so good about you ending up in the well?" "Well," said the second, "if you hadn't thrown me in, I certainly would have been a tasty morsel for the cannibals!"

(3) The law of retribution. Every wrong action or transgression brings its own punishment. Punishment does not come from God; it is a reaction to a bad action. So, the person who cheats and lies, cheats only himself; for example, the boy who cried wolf. As children, we were taught that cheaters never win. The law of karma states that cheaters will live lives of fear and worrying and that, in the end, they are the ones being cheated. This is true of most people who live in a culture of criminality; they are constantly fearful of being robbed or killed. Retribution for their actions is always nearby. Among Mafia-styled families, this proves to be particularly true; for they are prey of the law-enforcement agencies as well as other criminal forces.

(4) The law of resistance. Since most men are a composite of both good and not-so-good karma, they face resistance instilled by poor habits, which hinder the establishment of better ones. With the first attempts, it is natural for the aspirant to falter in setting up a system of good habits. However, through consistent practice, he will undoubtedly succeed. Habits are not innate.

Man has a free will to alter his life, and, although it requires great strength to do, it can be done. Simply, the laws of karma say, "We all make our own bed." It is time to take responsibility for who we are and refuse to be led anymore by our indulgent and selfish notions. If we desire to use it, we have the power to change ourselves. Too often, the law of karma is seen as a negative philosophy. Many people feel many of India's problems occur as a result of the law of karma. They think the people are taught that they are intwined and knotted, thus are imprisoned by negative destiny. Alas, this is quite a misconception.

Dharma. There is no adequate English definition for dharma. Roughly, it means the way of righteousness, the path that brings support, elevation, and peace. Adharma is unrighteousness, the path of no support, ignorance, and pain. Obviously, people interested in pursuing a virtuous life strive in the way of dharma. Dharma is an inner state of being, and it results from increasing good actions, such as are exemplified in the moral and ethical codes of the yamas and niyamas. I might add, nothing of any substance can be accomplished in yoga without being established in the path of righteousness. Dharma should not be viewed as "good" and adharma as "bad." Rather, dharma is the path of knowledge, adharma of ignorance. If one is leading a correct life, he is naturally established on the path of dharma. Adharmic qualities, as a result, fall away.

Swadharma. Swadharma is one's duties in accordance to the gunas, the qualities of nature. Following one's swadharma means that each person is great in his or her own way. We can all realize this if we understand and recognize our respective duties and perform them. Once we understand what we are supposed to do in this world, we can then simply go ahead and do it. The work-related fear, worry, and anxiety that accompany so many jobs are not there for the person who rests in his or her swadharma. Discharging responsibilities in a dispassionate way may well seem alien to a Western mind; the benefits, however, of this practice have been extolled by others for thousands of years. Imagine if heads of state, corporate executives, military leaders performed their duties in a dispassionate manner without the accompaniment of political games or intrigues. Imagine if parents and children knew exactly what their duties were. Since America, in particular, and Western society, in general, are still in the midst of various significant cultural revolutions, we are constantly living in a state of flux so that the definitions of responsibility are ever changing. There is nothing permanent and clear to grasp. Women, men, and children do not know what they should do. Discerning "what to do" is oftentimes a lifetime activity for some people. All their energies are absorbed in determining a simple common decision. Often, they are swayed by other people and either are attracted to, or repulsed by, the advice they receive. They run from their family's suggestions, only to be attracted to those of their friends. When they change friends and groups, they alter their goals as well. Until, at the end of their life, they see only a pattern of indecisiveness and inconclusion; motivated by a vague feeling of discontent. The scriptures say it is better to do your own duty poorly than someone else's well. The reverse of this form of thinking appears to be prevalent in this country. Successful men and women become unhappy in their work; searching in vain, they move on from one thing to another. Contrast contemporary life with the following little narrative.

As the story is told, there was once a great yogi who lived alone, deep in the forest. After many years of successful meditation, he achieved great powers. One day, while sitting in meditation, a crane flew over him and excreted on his head. He became furious and his thoughts immediately rose up and burned the bird to a crisp. He was quite pleased to find he had such an extraordinary gift and decided to go into town to explore further his newfound powers. He went in and, as was the custom of yogis in India, waited outside the door of a householder for alms. In response to his call, a woman, in hushed tones, replied, "Swami, please wait. I'll be right with you." But he grew angry and annoyed at being kept waiting by this "lowly woman." Just as his thoughts were reaching a feverish pitch, she called out, "Don't think that I, like the crane, can be extinguished so quickly." In utter surprise, he stopped, "Madam, how did you know that happened?" She explained, "I do not know any yoga asanas, nor do I even meditate, but I serve my sick husband with faith and devotion. In fact, I was with him when you came. I treat him as God personified, and I serve him accordingly. From this service, I have developed some small powers, though I never use them selfishly. If you really want to hear about the spiritual life, go see the butcher in the heart of the market place." The swami thanked her and went in search of the butcher. When he arrived at the village, he came upon a large crowd of people in the square, waiting for meat. In the midst of the crowd was a rough and burly-looking man, hacking away at slabs of beef, while constantly arguing with his customers. Could this be the man, the swami thought, the woman wanted me to meet and speak to? I can't believe it. Just as he was about to walk away, the butcher said, "Wait just one minute, Swamiji, I will be with you after I finish attending to my customers. I know the woman sent you." Again the yogi was dumbfounded at having his thoughts read. After all of the customers were taken care of, he accompanied the butcher back to his house. The butcher lived with his elderly parents, whom he waited on with great kind and loving care. After the man finished his familial duties, he sat down and held satsang—spiritual discussion—with the swami. The swami had never heard such beautiful and erudite descriptions of the scriptures. "How did you acquire this wonderful spiritual gift?" asked the swami. "I have done nothing special; I simply serve my family and my mother and father with sincere devotion." "But you are a butcher," the swami said, still incredulous at how this gift was attained. "It is a family business," he said, "which was given to me, and I perform it as my duty, my swadharma, dispassionately."

I do not necessarily maintain that all women should be devoted heart and soul to their husbands or that all men should assume their father's businesses; rather, I am saying that it is time we rethink about how we conceptualize and perform our duties. For it may not be just clergymen who "hear their calling," because those who rest in the knowledge of their swadharma *have* heard their call and have answered it. And in answering it, they have found their place in this world, be it great or small. In the great American dream, there seems to be a place for everyone who wants to be great. No one is striving to know his or her place; on the contrary, we are too often fighting what we think is destined. "Escaping the small town," "fleeing the big city," "getting out of the executive rat race," or "going to where the action is" are our ways of sometimes rationalizing away our life's duty. Many of us will be small, in order for a few to achieve greatness; but, in the eyes of the Lord, we should know that all are great in their own place. Real greatness comes to those who have realized that.

One final word about swadharma. Find out what you should be doing in this life and do it. Then devote all of your spiritual energies toward the task of self-realization. No lesser a person than Freud states: If neurotic energes are bound up in conflict, they cannot be freed for useful purposes. If we are constantly switching gears and being in a state of conflict, we cannot devote ourselves adequately to the spiritual task ahead.

The secret service. Secret service is action done with no thought toward reward. It refers specifically to good deeds. Not even a thank-you or a smile should be expected. It is in this sphere that selflessness is expanded, eventually to include all the actions of the individual. In other words, selfless service may originate in the context of a formal structure, i.e., a person doing charitable work for an organization. But as the individual progresses, he realizes selflessness can be found in every action performed. Anyone who has done charitable work, for example, seeing the joy on the faces of its recipients. Even more important, it teaches the individual that selflessness is applicable to all endeavors. Aside from teaching non-attachment to the fruits of our labor, selflessness teaches us equanimity of the mind. In our daily lives we perform both attractive and repugnant tasks. The whole premise of Karma yoga, however, is to rise above the very nature of work; in a sense, strike its very essence. It is the Lord's work, not our own we are performing; we are merely the instruments. So many people are concerned with whether they work in the country or the city. Others feel work should be interesting, or at least monetarily rewarding. Reasons such as these are definitely contrary to the spirit of Karma yoga. In this society, in which many of us pick and choose our jobs and life-styles, it is rare to find oneself in a situation where we do something "against our own will." That is why charitable work is so important; it teaches us to accept what is given. It may consist of low and menial tasks that, when executed with an even and balanced mind, reveal important lessons in selflessness. Once a great teacher visited our yoga institute. As he was climbing up the steps to the entrance, he came upon one of the disciples dutifully sweeping off the front stairs. He grabbed the broom from the young man and swept the stairs for him. True Karma yoga knows no status, no job descriptions, no discriminations. With a karma yogi, everything is his work because everything is His work.

Selfless service must be imbued with love for the individuals being served. They must be viewed as God personified and served accordingly. The individual with the capacity to serve with boundless love and dedication knows the secret of selfless service. So often people become functionaries or bureaucrats, serving in a mechanized and depersonalized manner. Such behavior is contrary to the spirit of selflessness. Every individual must be treated with equality, as if each were equally the most important person on the face of the earth.

Lastly, Karma yoga should be practiced quietly, without fanfare. Odious tasks are tests of one's dedication, not objects of avoidance. Praise should be borne as evenly as censure; and selfish pride has no home in the practice. If one person serves more people than another, it does not necessarily mean he or she is a "good" karma yogi. It is the quality of service that distinguishes the true karma yogi. The spirit of Karma yoga has been internalized when this quality of service extends to all and is inherent in all actions of the individual.

Pure selfishness. Karma yogis know that the greatest joy comes in service. They know that the entire world bows at the feet of a pure servant. For humanity is not only grateful for what it has received from the hand, but also from the heart. And it is this lesson that yoga gives to the world. Yogis are well aware that there is little that can be done to change the world. Yogis see the world as if it was a dog's curly tail. Every time someone tries to straighten it out, it snaps back. We try to eliminate poverty, but there are always some people poorer than others. We try to stamp out crime in one area, but yet it pops up in another. We finish one war, and we get ready for the next. The only way to alter the world is to change yourself, and *this* can be done through Karma yoga. All we do in the name of Karma yoga is, in essence, an attempt to change the practitioner. Again, that is why selflessness is selfish. In fact, there is no higher or purer selfishness than Karma yoga. For when individuals who are the recipients of your service see the joy you derive from the act, they and their attitudes change; they too begin to contemplate the spirit of selflessness and service and the joy that it brings. This is the only way the world can change and become harmonious in the practice of giving; from one, many; from many, the world.

Reincarnation. No talk on karma would be complete without discussing reincarnation. Yogis believe in the transmigration of the soul; this is the very core of their belief in the Karma yoga system. The sum total of karmas affect the next life an individual assumes. If the previous existence was virtuous, then the next one will be so too. If you have difficulty in believing about reincarnation, try to find a copy of *Twenty Cases Suggestive of Reincarnation*. It is a compilation of twenty recorded cases of individuals who remember their past lives without ever being told about them by anyone. If we look at people as separate individuals, we can see that reincarnation might explain some of the unanswered questions of scientists. For instance, different people have different tastes and temperaments. Why is this so? Why should members of the same family be so different? Even identical twins eventually go their separate ways. How often do we hear parents exclaim about a "wayward" child, "I really don't know where he came from. He doesn't think or act like us at all." Obviously environment and psychological makeup are not the only factors in shaping an individual's personality, character, and destiny. For if we can take two individuals from the same family, with the same background, we will see that they are sometimes more diverse than two individuals with different backgrounds. There must be an additional force that social scientists have not yet discovered; a force that is propelling all individuals along their own separate paths. It is said that we all walk to the beat of a different drummer; however, more correctly put, the beat may be different, but the drummer is the same. The beat is different because our capacity to hear it is different. These capacities did not just come to us full blown, already formed. Our capacities of the present were shaped by our actions in the past. What we are "here and now" is very much related to what happened "there and then."

In the universe there is nothing left up to chance. This may sound very fatalistic, but, in truth, it is not. Unfortunately, the laws of karma and reincarnation have received "bad publicity" over the years because of a fundamental misunderstanding about these laws and the concept of freedom. (For a fuller discussion of freedom, see the next chapter.) Westerners believe that the concept of karma has been responsible for the indolence and passivity of the Oriental world in general, and the Indian people specifically. Reincarnation does not induce passivity and indolence; it occurs as a result of all people having to work out their accumulated karma. A person may be passive, owing to former lifetimes of passivity; there will, however, come a time when the individual will reach his saturation point and start to move out of his mold.

The concept of reincarnation gives one a much broader perspective on the whole problem of human existence, because one sees that lifetimes have been spent in adharmic ways and will not yield quickly to overnight solutions like drugs or special techniques. Only when the individual gets to the point of taking on a spiritual practice can any thought be given to transcending these influences. Until then, freedom as we know it, is impossible. For there can be no freedom or free will while the individual is in the clutches of karmic influence. But the moment one intuits a way out and moves toward that direction, one begins to exercise free will. Then the motivation for the present actions are not wholly dictated by the previous ones. Thus, the closer the aspirant moves toward the selfless ideal, the more he realizes that he is just an instrument of the Lord's Will, a channel for spirituality to become manifested on this planet. At this point, the disciple has no desires of his own, and he may experience a deep sense of freedom. "Freedom is another word for nothing left to lose," says the song. And so it is for the yogi who has reached this elevated state of consciousness. For him, the rounds of rebirth and death are over, the karmic cycle has stopped. But still, for the realized yogi, he stays in the world; because although there may not be anything personal left to do, the Lord has jobs for His servants.

chapter six — Real Work, Getting Down to It

The commitment.

No discussion pertaining to practices can really be complete without saying something about the nature of freedom and discipline. Primary to all the practices we've talked about is the premise that they can lead the practitioner to freedom. That the practices require discipline often puts beginning students in a quandary. For the two terms, discipline and freedom, appear on the surface to be contradictory. How can one be free in the midst of control? Often, this conflict produces an emotional strain, affecting the student's practices. As I've said before, nothing can be gained on the yogic path without real work. Yoga practice, as in any other endeavor, means an all-out commitment to real work. That is why I gave the practice chapters headings signifying various different types of work. I did not want anyone to get the wrong idea, that the practices are light and breezy. Instead, I wanted the titles to spell out individual commitment to the practices; only in that way can real progress be made.

What is freedom?

It is a state of being free; free from those bonds which keep us from realizing ourselves. Freedom is also spontaneity, synchronicity. It is knowing what to do at any moment, and doing it. Freedom, however, is not running away from responsibilities. Being spontaneous does not imply dodging one's duty. After all, can you really run away from your problems? Wherever you go, problems follow; they are part of the mind. Freedom is not immoderation. Allowing your senses to run loose, going to excesses without restraints, is not freedom. The greatest bondage that the immoderate person faces is his attachment to abandonment. When an individual is really free, he is able to free himself from the life-style of immoderation. The immoderate individual does not realize to what extent he has limited his freedom. He is unaware that his spontaneity and his freedom have been directly dependent upon circumstances of indulgence.

What is discipline?

Discipline is control. There are two basic types of discipline: external and internal.

External discipline. External control leads to internal control of the mind. Like sandbags on the banks of a flooding river, control is necessary to focus the mind and keep it from spilling into extraneous areas. We know that a river, whose banks have broken down, spreads out and loses its power. The same river, with a barrier fortifying its banks, flows down with an increased intensity and control. If one controls the mind, through the disciplines, the mind has power to focus and cuts deep into the underlying reality. Without control, the mind widens out, superficially moving from one thought to another. In order to begin developing this power, one must learn to detach the mind from sense-objects, and attach it to the underlying spiritual practice. For example, the practices of karma yoga lead you from the actual task of washing a floor, to the spiritual truth that you are nothing more than an extension of the mop you hold. Like the mop, you are being used by the consciousness for its purpose and not your own. In all of the external disciplines, you detach a portion of the mind from the specific discipline and attach it to the underlying spiritual practice. Teachers, in referring to japa, like to relate the humorous example of the wife, who while caring for the home she shares with her husband, thinks of her boyfriend while doing her chores. So, like the wife, the spiritual seeker, although engaged in his worldly (external) duties, always keeps a portion of his mind occupied on the spiritual practice or proper attitude.

Internal discipline. External discipline leads to internal discipline. Thus, as you perform the practices, you are concurrently establishing an internal strength. With this strength you are strong and stable enough to withstand temptations, like a candle flame that, in the midst of a windy place, remains steady. After several years of practice, a student will find his internal discipline able to stand alone, without aid from the external, or even internal, practice. However, in the beginning, all aspirants must stick close, and bind themselves to their practices; for without this initial binding, one cannot establish internal discipline. One must take refuge in the practices, as one's source and salvation.

Freedom and discipline.

Many people view discipline as a repressive force and freedom as an unlimited license. The truth is, we all have discipline in our lives and do not, on the whole, react to it as a subverting power. In order to execute or complete any task, one must be moderately disciplined. As children, we were disciplined, or trained, not to soil our clothing and to use the toilet. Also, if we were bad, we were disciplined to act according to our parents' expectations. We all admire great athletes, but certainly their accomplishments are the results of disciplined lives of self-control and will power. The conquest of Mount Everest by Sir Edmund Hillary (and Tenzing Norkay) is such an example of a great disciplined mind. And yogis, too, are no different. Difficulty arises when new aspirants feel they must deny themselves, limit their choices, and curtail their freedoms, in establishing themselves on the disciplined path. The trouble is not the control but rather the conception of freedom. In America, we define freedom to mean independence of choice. Thus, if one has the freedom to choose where he lives, what kind of job he has, and what kind of lifestyle he maintains, an American essentially believes he is free. Two hundred years have passed since the founding of this country, and there are still people unable to exercise their freedom of choice. Many dissident minority groups voice the feeling that they have been manipulated by the system and denied this right. It is unfortunate that this concept of liberty so thoroughly permeates the American and the Western mind, for it really has so little to do with freedom of choice. To be spontaneous and at peace with oneself, no matter the situation, is freedom. Why man must involve himself in areas he has no control over will always remain a mystery. Perhaps man's intelligence is his greatest curse, as well as his greatest boon. No matter who you are, the controls you have over your choices or their quality are very little. In the great restaurant of the universe, man is always trying to increase the choices on the menu. He seems to forget he has come to the restaurant to eat, and make a selection, not to increase the offerings. One's energy should be used in selecting the proper choice, the choice of dharma. The choices that lead to freedom are given to everyone. It is just that we foolishly wish to increase our choices, thus further confusing the issue. Disciplined existence fits perfectly within the realm of choices. We all love nature, with its purity and freedom. Let's look at a tree; it doesn't have anywhere near as much freedom of choice as we have. Its life plan is given to it; an oak tree cannot become a sycamore nor will a palm tree grow in New York City. A tree's life is disciplined and dependent upon its environment. And with that discipline, it exists in relative harmony within its surroundings. It behaves as it was trained, to be a tree. Though this may sound oversimplified, I believe that nature has many of the answers to man's existential problems. Within nature lies the model for us to follow. The tree exists without many choices. It leads a disciplined life. But yet, it exists as a real and viable part of nature's scheme. It lives as both a separate entity and a unit of the forest matrix. Like people, no two trees are exactly alike; they may be the same species, but they are not the same. So freedom implies the ability to express one's inimitable potential, but, without the tree's inherent discipline, or nature's, for that matter, the oak or the sycamore would not realize its true self. Without parameters of control, the essence would not be manifested.

Coping with cop-outs.

Knowing what to do, yet not doing it, is a common problem for spiritual aspirants. If we understand that discipline is needed for freedom to manifest, we can begin to deal with the inevitable cop-outs that result from our attempts in establishing the practices. Newer students usually have an initial burst of enthusiasm which very soon cools off. Old habits soon reappear. At this point, the aspirant is faced with the task of overcoming his former karma. Rationalizations crop up whenever behavior is at odds with the practices. The spiritual seeker is in a turmoil; he realizes, for the first time, the enormity of the task, as he finds himself confronted with the reality of his life. Reality brings pain because it has destroyed the aspirant's expectations and attachments. Old methods, like copping-out, are brought into play to deal with the pain. Psychologists state that everyone regresses, and, if done in moderation, it is a healthy maneuver for the individual. Copping-out is a form of regression and a natural and healthy thing to do, *if* not carried too far. Usually, during any real major conflict with the practices, or the teacher, these cop-outs and rationalizations can be dealt with and eventually stopped. The Law of Resistance is in effect here. (See Karma yoga section.) This is the very reason the old habits will reappear. These old habits, or mental attitudes, vie with the new ones for control. Regularity in the practices, as a result, will swing precariously in the balance. One rationalization frequently brought into play is freedom of choice. The mind will use any concept to maintain its control and power over the individual. And if we understand that freedom of choice is just that, a concept, and not actually freedom, then we can deal, at least intellectually, with the whole idea of copping-out. Rationalizations result from other causes too. The aspirant must open his or her consciousness to examination and ask, "Is my mind reacting this way because I have pushed it too hard?" or "Is it rebelling and reacting this way because I have given it too much leeway?" If you have honestly confronted the problem, you know there is a third question to be asked, "What kind of person am I?" The latter should produce an objective analysis of your major personality characteristics. Are you an energetic and highly motivated individual, or a lazy and lethargic person? Your response to this question will bear weight on your answer to the first two. For example, if you feel you've been pushing yourself and, in your "heart of hearts," know yourself to be an irresponsible individual, the former is most likely a rationalization. Or, if you are an overly conscientious person, and feel you have given your mind too much leeway, it is quite probable that you have been pushing too hard. The common reason for the mind to cop-out is because it either tries too hard, or not hard enough. Beginning students usually either whip their minds into turmoils of distraction or allow them to sit in pools of stagnation. Once you've discovered which is your particular problem, the solution is relatively simple.

Keeping schedules.

The solution to both lax and compulsive spiritual behavior is the same. Regularity in one's sadhana, practice, is an absolute necessity. Practices must be ordered and done in a reasonable manner. Composing schedules may be a distasteful task to the lax individual, but they're an invaluable tool in helping one live in a disciplined manner. The schedule should not be made too difficult. In the beginning, meditation periods should not be very long, nor should an entire day be spent doing Hatha yoga. It is better to integrate the practices into your life, rather than to drastically change your life to encompass only the practices. Slow, steady infusions of the practices into your routine will lessen the chances of a difficult situation occurring for either you or the people around you. The slow and steady approach also provides some practical exercises in self-control for the overzealous student. The new student should commence his practices with short periods of meditation in the morning, upon awakening, and in the evening prior to retiring. Hatha yoga can be done at either of the above times, though it may be more advisable for the novice to perform the postures in the evening if the body is especially stiff. Beginning periods of meditation should be no longer than thirty to forty-five minutes in the morning and fifteen minutes in the evening. Practice Hatha yoga for fifteen to thirty minutes. This slow regimen can be increased gradually over a time span of three to six months. As in the practices of Hatha yoga, nothing should be pushed or forced; you should feel comfortable in doing whatever practices you have decided upon. You are not in competition; therefore, the length of time other people spend meditating or doing asanas is not your concern. Examine yourself and your abilities, and within your capacities, do the practices for reasonable periods of time. After the short regimen has become established in your daily routine, additional practices can be included, such as scriptural study, chanting, mantra writing (the writing of one's mantra 108 times). Don't take on more than you can handle. Mauna, fasting (on a regular basis), and tradak can be added one, two, or three times, spread out during the space of a week. There is no end to the amount of practices you can add; much depends on the time you have. But remember, if you place your expectations too high, you may become disappointed if you fail to reach them. If you do begin to cop-out, you can discipline yourself by fasting an extra day, or depriving yourself of some treat, thereby doing extra practices to compensate for the neglected ones. Learn to be your own good parent; don't let yourself "get away with murder," yet don't be too hard on yourself, either. Good parents train their children with firmness, not destructiveness. Some people believe self-discipline to mean some kind of masochism or mental flagellation. This is not true. You must learn to be beneficent when you have done something admirably and punish yourself when you have done something disgraceful. If you have done the spiritual practices well, reward yourself. Through the years of schedules, one can develop the facilities to turn within and view oneself objectively.

Associations.

Shankaracharya said, "One of the immediate benefits of cultivating good associations is that you find that you are not in bad company." Good associations are those people who lead virtuous lives and give you support for leading one too. Bad company are those individuals who live lives which are adharmic, non-virtuous, and who desire you to conduct yourself in a similar manner. Indifferent company comprise those people whose lives are not particularly virtuous, but they will not stop you from "doing your thing." In the beginning of spiritual practice, it is common for the new aspirant to fence himself off and strictly cultivate good associations. The young aspirant, like the newly planted seedling, can easily be destroyed by outside forces, unless protected by a fence of sorts. That is why some people choose to live in a protected environment, like an ashram. (See next chapter.) Keeping bad company can cause doubt about one's spiritual life, making it difficult to move ahead. These people may be anyone—friend, relative, or spouse. Separating oneself from bad associations is sometimes the new aspirant's most painful work. However, if you are serious about moving forward on the spiritual path, cutting these ties is an absolute necessity. If these relationships are kept intact and continued, they can only bring pain in the future. This may sound extreme, but what often occurs is that bad associations actively participate in keeping the aspirant from his practices. They not only keep up a steady propaganda campaign, but make it awkward to do the practices in their presence. If on the other hand, the individuals, whom you are with, are kind but not especially spiritual, they immediately are not detrimental to your study. I classify these people as indifferent. They do not lead virtuous lives, but they do not keep you from leading your life. In the beginning, these relationships are easy to deal with, but after a while, even their presence may cause doubt and affect your progress on the path. It should be understood that there are no such people as "bad people." This term is used by insecure people to feel superior. We use the terms good and bad here to effectively simplify matters. Bad people are not bad, though they may be to some degree misguided. But because of their relative ignorance of spiritual life, one should try to avoid their company when first starting out on the path. Be aware that "good people," too, may not be completely good. Their motives, at times, may be less than pure. The evangelizing yogi is a prime example. Usually, this missionary is a new convert to yoga, who is so consumed with the magnitude of his experiences that he is incapable of understanding why everyone isn't doing the practices. They would like to believe that yoga has completely changed their lives, but in truth, these people haven't yet shed their old skins. Their manners and attitudes are still tainted with their former life-styles. So be aware of the self-righteous person, no matter who he is.

Separation from past associations.

Freeing yourself from bad or indifferent associations poses some difficulty. First, you must deal with your own attachments to these people and the life you shared with them. There are two basic ways this separation occurs. The first is to sever or drastically limit the old relationship. The second is to slowly draw yourself out of the relationship. The latter is infinitely more painful, for the conflict is prolonged. In the former, the pain may be acute, but it is over relatively quickly. Once you have freed yourself from your attachments to people and former lives, you still must extricate yourself from others' attachments to you, and this, indeed, is a much more arduous task. Friends and relatives may hold on to you long after you have changed and even physically left their presence. As long as this former life retains its ties, there may be some difficult moments in your progress. But gradually, as people realize you have changed, and are not coming back to your former ways, their relationship to you will subsequently alter. The various changes that occur when you move from one life-style to another must be done with great care and understanding toward the people they affect. The best way to cope during this difficult transitional period is by maintaining close and constant contact with people who are of your like mind. Their support is important to your practice.

Backsliding.

Backsliding in spiritual practices is inevitable. You will learn to expect it and use it as a source for future progress. It is usually caused by (1) recurrence of old habits, (2) bad associations, (3) irregularity of practices, and (4) overconfidence. These are usually manifestations of the cosmic rationalization. This rationalization permits backsliding to occur in the name of "freedom." Keep a close watch on the cosmic rationalization, and learn to recognize it in yourself. Rationalizations are the hardest mind deceptions to catch. Chances are you will be fooled innumerable times, but persevere and return to your disciplines; the mind will eventually stop its tricks. Regard your practices as if they were your mantra; constantly bring yourself back to them when you wander away. It is the process of taking oneself back to the practices that stops backsliding and firmly establishes the practitioner as an internally disciplined individual. Like a baby who is first introduced to candy, the mind may not like the practices on first viewing, but once it has tasted the sweetness the practices bring, it will not only like it but return for more. Once you have internal discipline, you can move with confidence into difficult, non-spiritual realms. However, you should be wary of feeling over-confident, for spiritual development takes time, and it is not helpful to your progress to be "cocky" about what you have attained. Like film that is being processed, it must be in the developer a certain length of time. If you take the negatives out too soon, they will be ruined. So it is with the spiritual seeker. If the seeker exposes himself to the world and its hostile environment too soon, his spiritual life will be ruined. People do not become yogis overnight. The goal of a true yogi is more than a nice smile, or a peaceful feeling. These are certainly nice things to have; the point is, they only achieve permanence after a long time of devoted practice. Yogis, like doctors or lawyers, must spend years in preparing themselves. Backsliding is a good indicator of how far the seeker has spiritually developed. Without backsliding, he never knows what areas need further work. Without it, he never knows the rationalizing and conniving capabilities of his mind. With yoga, and the steady disciplines, we can all discover the inner reality of the mind and go beyond its selfish nature.

part three

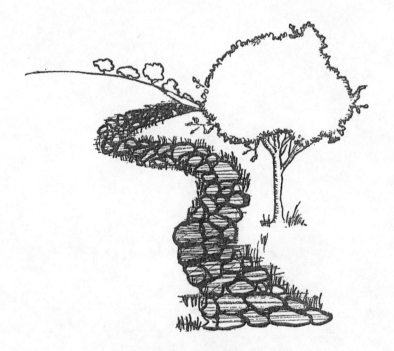

on the
way out

chapter one – Communes, Communities, and the Real World

In the previous chapter, I discussed the necessity of associating with good company. Now, I would like to continue and delve into the various types of supportive groups one can join as a beginning aspirant. Almost all of us need some supportive group, be it family, friends, or fellow workers. Such is the case for the spiritual seeker too. To put it succinctly, "There is strength in numbers." Groups help you get over the difficult transitional period when you are discarding one life for another. Group members provide the knowledge of their experiences; and with their assistance, problems can be avoided or at least shared. They help you maintain your balance, providing you with a proper perspective on your new situation. Frequently, having divorced himself from family and friends, the beginning student has no one but the spiritual group to turn to. Thus, for some people, it is necessary to move in and live among their spiritual brothers and sisters, while for others, occasional visiting with them is sufficient. It depends basically on the individual and his involvement. Whatever the degree of involvement, support is offered in many ways; it can be psychological and emotional, as well as spiritual. Speaking from my own experience, I cannot overemphasize their importance to, or their necessity for, the beginning spiritual seeker.

Communes.

In our society alone, there seem to be as many varieties of communes as there are people to belong to them. There are political communes, gay communes, psychological therapy communes; there are communes with hundreds of people, and there are communes with four or five people. Some are composed of families, some of single people; others are mixtures of the two. Some are loosely cohesed; others are strictly ruled. Some are situated in the country hills, others in the city slums. Amid the myriad choices sits the yoga ashram. In India, ashrams are monasteries. However, in the United States, the term yoga ashram is applied to a variety of spiritual communes. Though a few American yoga ashrams function as monasteries, most commune ashrams are loosely run, with single, married, and family people living in them. The shape of the ashram, and what actually goes on there, depends largely on the basic philosophy of the ashram's leader. If an ashram doesn't have a leader, it is most likely a loosely run affair. Indian ashrams almost always have leaders or, at least, sets of principles to guide the ashramites.

What to look for. If you are planning to join a yoga commune, it is advisable to visit it first and speak to the people who have been there for a relatively long time. Only in this manner can you sense how the community functions. Try to speak to the spiritual leader to find out if you can live up to the principles he or she sets. Survey the ashram's physical surroundings. Is it dirty and scattered or clean and ordered? Simple things tell you an enormous amount about the community. Physical reality is at the crux of most teachings of yoga. Consider very strongly whether the community is of a practical bent. Read everything you can about the place; stay there as a guest for a few days;

participate in the schedule. In India, moving into an ashram traditionally means the individual has accepted the principles of the leader and has become, in a sense, a formalized student of the teacher. This is a reasonable expectation of any ashram. It is improper to move into an ashram under any other circumstances. If you have doubts about the spiritual practices of that commune, visit frequently, until your questions have been answered one way or another.

The importance of a leader. No ashram should be without a leader. A grouping of friends does not make an ashram. In fact, unless there is a teacher present, the ashram will probably have many problems. Participatory democracy is usually not found in a yoga ashram. What the teacher says, goes. And it must be this way, for the teacher is responsible for the spiritual life of the students. His decision, even if it concerns the most personal matters of the individual's life, must be obeyed. This unilateral power is what makes life in a yoga ashram interesting as well as difficult. It is in the ashram that the teacher really works on the student, and within this relationship, the student learns about himself. People may come and go and only see the nice side of the teacher; however, it is only the students who see and feel the firey side which burns them regularly. Living with the teacher is usually strenuous. Sometimes the teacher feasts the students one day and fasts them the next. In some ashrams, the students work almost continuously, with barely any time set aside for meditation or other practices. At times, a yoga ashram may seem like nothing less than a lunatic asylum. Actually, Sivananda once made such a comparison. "Look at my disciples," he said. "They run around, all dressed in white or orange; is there any real difference between this and an asylum? They're really like the people in the asylum; they're good for nothing aside from practicing yoga. Well, at least like the asylum, we keep them off the street." But as crazy as a yoga ashram may superficially appear, it is a very peaceful and holy place underneath. If you find this, you know you have come upon a real ashram, with a real teacher directing it. It is inconsequential whether the teacher is physically present, three thousand miles away, or has passed away;

what does matter is that the teachings live on within the students.

Life realities. Life in the ashram is not an easygoing, carefree existence. I mention this first because it is better to be prepared and familiar with the possible difficulties of this kind of life before entering an ashram. Your privacy will be invaded; your personal preferences will be ignored; your individuality will be obscured; and your pride will be trampled upon. You will do fine if you understand and accept these aspects before coming to the ashram. Few people, however, are fully prepared for the experience that awaits them. You live in close quarters, sometimes with many people, all having different habits, perceiving things from their own separate worlds. And to come together and form a cohesive, individualized group is a very difficult task. During the formative stages of a group, conflicts are just about inevitable, and until the ashram becomes established, these rough moments will continue to reoccur. If you are the type of person who would rather avoid such situations, I recommend joining a well-established ashram, where the power struggles have long since worn themselves out. For until a yoga ashram is established, people expend an inordinate amount of time and energy in vying for power. Even the presence of a leader or a teacher cannot stop these struggles. They are the reality of any commune, spiritual groups notwithstanding. (See the extended spiritual community below.)

Economic realities. Almost all of the communes and yoga ashrams I know of have had some economic difficulties. Most of these ashrams, born of the counterculture movement of the 60s, eschewed the whole area of financial responsibility. They soon found that, if they wanted to put together a viable commune, a steady income was necessary. Most of the ashrams were founded by young people, without established careers, who had little, if any, financial experience. Periodic economic upheavals were a common occurrence in a number of communes. Therefore, before entering a yoga ashram, familiarize yourself thoroughly with its financial condition. Be wary of a commune that permits you to move in without requiring some show of financial responsibility on your part. The ashram is unstable and probably will prove to be an unsatisfactory experience. Look for an ashram that has set economic guidelines, that are followed by the community at large. Of course, as a member, you will have to actively participate in supporting the commune. Various ashrams have outside business which employ their members. And some ashram members work in the outside community as well. Some ashrams allow their members to keep some money; in others, everyone pools his entire monetary assets. Either way, the choice should always be yours; that is why it is important to visit the ashram before you commit yourself.

A final note: If you're doubtful about your commitment in an ashram, look for one in which you are permitted to retain some of your personal money. This will avoid the occurrence of any future unpleasant situations. Whatever type of ashram you may move into, expect to be a financial link in its supporting mechanism.

Group discipline. People frequently move into a yoga ashram for this particular aspect. A great deal of support can be derived from this form of discipline. Rising early, and meditating, is much easier in a group than by yourself. When individuals jointly do their practices, they progress to a group level. In other words, new students are aided by the more experienced ones, and are brought up quickly to the shared level of the group. This is a prime reason why the continuity and integrity of group discipline must be maintained. In the beginning, you may discover the group discipline to be very supportive; but after a while, you may desire to escape its regimentation. Remember, the discipline is not your enemy; it is (through group practices) assisting you in becoming established on the path. That, after all, is your primary goal in moving into the yoga ashram. Therefore, when you visit a yoga ashram, be sure to look at the level of discipline. Assess realistically whether you can live in, and benefit from, its environment.

Structure. All ashrams have a different structure. Some are comprised of families; some have none. Some are more monastic than others. Some are highly disciplined, and others are not. Be conscious of their variations. One is not better than another; each answers the needs of different particular people.

Communities, the satsang group.

This type of spiritual community is a fellowship of people who frequently meet for spiritual discussions. (Institutionalized religions are satsang groups on a large scale.) Those people who attend these groups usually do not desire the close, confining discipline or commitment of a commune or yoga ashram. These groups meet periodically; they conduct spiritual discussions which serve as the focal point for the community. Also, on occasion, they meet for other social functions. They are located wherever people find the need for them. The forms they take are as varied as the environments they reside in. Some spiritual groups have set up planned spiritual communities. One such organized community, set up by the disciples of Paramahamsa Yogananda, is the Ananda Cooperative Community, located in Grass Valley, California. It is situated on a parcel of land, where the people work at small cottage industries, running the gamut from making incense to hand-carved wooden toys. Setting up such a community in the country is a very difficult task. It took a great deal of energy and dedication on the part of the founding members. Coping with the harsh economic realities of rural living is sometimes the main concern of the spiritual community of that locale, and until these problems are settled, the community is not really established. Like the commune, the spiritual community asks more of its members than a desire to live in the country. Other rurally located spiritual communities may not be as highly organized as the Ananda group. For example, a community has evolved around the Satchidananda Ashram in Connecticut. The involved individuals bought and rented houses in the vicinity of the spiritual center. They do not own any businesses together; rather, most are employed in the surrounding community. Not all spiritual communities form around a particular spiritual center or institute. Some exist for the mere communion between members. This is true of the followers of the late Kirpal Singh. These spiritual communities usually appear to be the providences of married couples and families, while communes and yoga ashrams are best suited for single people. The close communal life in the ashram aids individual discipline. It allows the single people to develop free from distractions. The more open atmosphere of the communities is conducive to family life. But even the communities are supportive of the individual seeker. To facilitate change, the community subtly exerts pressures on the individual. After all, if one moves into a community of yogis, it will be less likely that he will engage in his former habits, than if he lived in a twenty-five-story high-rise in Manhattan. Community sanction exists and is very real; that is one reason why individuals move into such communities.

The extended spiritual community. The spiritual community, by definition, is open-ended; a place where people can share ideas. City satsang groups exemplify this ideal. Usually, people are introduced to the spiritual practices through a member of the community. If a spiritual community is to maintain its vitality, it should always be ready to extend itself to new people who introduce new ideas. New energy also brings problems; sometimes members become entrenched in their ways and balk at any attempts the new members may make in changing things. Older adherents sometimes feel the new members lack respect and understanding, and these people, in turn, feel the older ones are on power trips. Conflict ensues, and the community stands still. All groups, whether spiritual or not, fall prey to infighting and power struggles. This, alas, is the nature of bringing people together. Therefore, this problem must be solved before the group evolves to its second phase.

This stage is a time of close community involvement, when everyone is united; a very special love relationship unfolds. The community, however, cannot rest at this stage; it must go further or else, again, become stale and close-mind. "Group-think" will evolve, with the members expending their energies validating their own points of view. New members entering this very heady environment will very likely discard their dissention and their individuality. Many spiritual communities, particularly communes, fall into this phase of group evolution. The group exudes a feeling of self-satisfaction; suffering and fighting have disappeared from its midst. But in a very real way, this is not true. The group, however, must pass through yet one more phase. Acceptance is the key word of this stage: acceptance of people, regardless of their tastes or temperaments, and acceptance of criticism, not as a judgment, but as an assistance. Such would be a spiritual community that has evolved to its fullest. It is one where new members can be accepted for what they are and not for what they might be. Obviously, it is most advantageous for anyone contemplating a spiritual group, to do so when and if it has reached this phase.

Spiritual groups, like any others, disperse and die. When the world of the community is finished, it dissolves. There should be no unpleasant feelings when this occurs. For a moment in time a group comes together, its members learn what they can from each other, then part and go their separate ways, to transmit their knowledge to others. To hold on to any one in particular for the mere sake of maintaining it, is a very deep and destructive attachment. We use groups for our evolution and development. From the moment of our birth, to our last breath, we move from one group to another. All of these group experiences enrich us and aid in our growth. The length of our memberships vary from group to group, depending upon our interest, involvement, and the potential for real growth. Groups exist as long as the members feel the above three factors are being met. It is useless for group members to hold onto a group's existence when these functions are no longer there.

The real world.

Sometimes it is difficult to determine when the time is right to leave the spiritual community or commune and move out on your own. After living for months or years in one of these communities, the world can look both frightening and awesome. With the proper perspective, this frightening, "insane" place can be seen as a real home. When a yogi evolves to the point where he no longer needs a protected environment, he can move anywhere, among anyone; for everywhere is his home, and everyone is his family. This self-assuredness comes as a result of years of spiritual practices. There is an urge to move out into the world, from within. At the proper time, and in the proper way, circumstances provide the door to your leaving. Living in the real world does not necessitate your being a full-blown yogi. However, if one is to live an unwavering life of a yogi in the "real" world, one must first go through the preliminary steps. Each life situation presents its own particular problems. For single people, temptations are constantly cropping up in the world that would not be present in a sheltered environment. For the family, the problems are different, though nevertheless as numerous. Children, not raised in a protected, spiritual atmosphere, tend to rebel against their parents' spirituality. Though rebellion occurs in most families, the attractions of the outside world appear exceptionally enticing when the family life is so different. If a spiritual person is attempting to train his children in a particular way of life, an overnight stay at a friend's house can be fraught with temptation and peril. The violence in the games and behavior of young children is extremely upsetting to the spiritual family. Living in the world definitely puts one's beliefs to the test. When you leave the spiritual community, you must transform your home into the very center of your worship. In a sense, it becomes your protected area, your sanctuary. If you are conscious of the pitfalls present in the world, you can take sufficient precautionary measures to avoid or deal with these inevitable problems. That is why a home is so important; it helps keep your practices intact and provides you with a working base. No matter how bad things get, there is always solace and comfort at home. However, if your home is a shambles, you have obviously not established the yogic spirit there; life then can be like riding the high seas in a rudderless boat. Once you have set your house in order, you are prepared to learn the lessons the world has to offer.

The world as your teacher.

It is not only the well-experienced old-timer who claims to be a graduate from the school of hard knocks; most people seem to characterize their relationships with the world in that manner. There is hardly a person who can float through the worldly maze unscathed. In fact, it takes a great deal of courage to open oneself up to the experiences and teachings of the world. Aside from courage, an individual must have stability. The world is a testing ground; it gives all its inhabitants an exam in living, every day. Particular problems reoccur daily. New situations present new areas to work on. Sometimes in frustration, people try to run away and hide from their problems. They fail to realize that the difficulties they are having are firmly rooted in their minds.

Some people seek the sanctity of a yoga ashram, but even there, the world reaches in. Now, yoga neither hides you nor helps you flee from the world's vicissitudes. It does, however, prepare you for the world's tests. Good yoga ashrams and communities understand the necessity of facing the world openly. They make a point of dealing with its challenges, as they come, day by day.

The world is fickle, sometimes good and other times bad. Sometimes there is prosperity, other times, famine. The world is the dualistic playground of God, and man is the ball being tossed from side to side. If you go within, and have a central point to focus on, this dualism is mirrored in your soul. You are the pivot of the fluctuation. Some days you are excited, other days depressed. Sometimes you want everything and other times nothing. This crazy seesaw living is normal for most people. But a yogi's life sees more of the world than this. In a sense, life is like a boat riding the rapids, constantly being on guard not to let in any water. A boat filled with water sinks below the surface, tossed deep and hard by the currents within. You must step beyond the comings and goings of both the external world and your internal psyche. The world says, "I am beautiful; I am ugly"; you are attracted by one and repulsed by the other. In a sense, the guru is like that also; one side is loving and gentle, the other side, raging and fierce. But all the time he is saying, Look within; look beyond this form; see what is really there. And all the time the world is secretly saying, too, Look within; my punishments and rewards should only cause you to go within and discover who you are in my ever-changing environment. To know yourself is to know the world. Once you learn to see the world as your teacher, you will come to love its strange and beautiful dance. Pain, too, will be a true ally, as Sivananda said, "Pain is my friend; come on pain!"; and pleasures will be regarded as transitory, fleeting moments. And someday you will wonder in awe at God's plaything: this incredible, mystical world.

Humanity as your family.

Sometimes living in a closed environment like a yoga ashram can produce a kind of xenophobia, where one tends to view the outside world in threatening stereotypes. Living in the world provides the chance to develop a sense of spirituality toward people. People are not all evil and adharmic; rather, they are striving for their own divinity. With this vision, you know even the most displaced and confused individual is stumbling toward self-knowledge. The feeling of "oneness" results from this awareness of other's divinity. In essence, we are all of one spiritual family, no matter what external or internal differences exist. Once one abides in that spirit, then those differences are like specs of dust. But even though these differences will not be emphasized, they should be recognized. For example, in a family, the father does not switch roles with the son, nor the mother with the daughter. We all have our parts to play in life. It is in these roles that we realize greatness. Greatness, though, does not come from the statements and perceptions of your fellow man. It is seen and appreciated solely through the eyes of the Lord. Most truly great people are unrecognized as such by the rest of humanity. The truly gentle people, the upholders of dharma, are the ones who are most often the neglected members of society. It appears that society would rather publicize and propagandize the adharmic individual. Once we realize our respective roles, we will see, through our cleared minds, the rest of the family of man struggling to realize theirs. We feel compassion for their struggle and will help in any way we can. Some people misconstrue this attitude and feel that it is a license to open your doors to anyone that wants to come in. This is not quite true. Not everyone out in the world is that pure. You must take care that your home, and your mind, are not disturbed by irritating influences. As you know your place and role, then you will make sure others also maintain theirs. There should be no discrimination as to personality, religion, ethnic, or racial standing in this stance. To do otherwise indicates a strong sense of insecurity in your own position. This attitude, which is easily discernible, will far from elicit the respect and understanding you originally desired. There is only one way to gain respect, and that is by giving it.

Yoga and society.

Many people believe yogis want nothing to do with societal changes. To say the very least, this is a misconception. Yoga practitioners strongly desire to affectively influence society; they desire to cause changes for the positive education and enlightenment of all the world's people. Yoga wants its basic universal message to dispel the distinctions of caste, color, creed, religion, and class. Yoga would like to see the distinctions between national states disintegrate. Yoga practices and teaches universal brotherhood in an all-encompassing manner. How can we be brothers if we exist within our own separate houses, each following our own particular beliefs? Yoga believes that these changes can be instituted by understanding each individual's particular nature. No laws can bring all the desired results one wants, for laws constantly alter as man's mind constantly changes. Laws are created, countries rise and fall, revolutions come and go, but man in his struggle to understand himself is still a mystery. People, with their riches, cannot buy away their misery, nor any law put an end to it. What country can remain vital if a large segment of its population remains ignorant and unhappy? Laws may raise economic standards, but it appears that as someone benefits on this earth, someone else loses. In America, we have built our great economic standard on the plundering of our, and other's, resources and the exploitation of our environment. Dissention erupts as our technology advances us and leaves other nations struggling behind. We provide for ourselves, oblivious to the more desperate needs of others around us. If there is some advanced planet out there and its inhabitants are looking upon us, they must think how primitive and silly we are, to rob and steal so mercilessly from each other and from our land. If we are to advance as a society or as a planet, we must realize the essential divinity of all people and initially express it in ourselves. Only through this expression will others receive the message and learn that there is more to life than the pursuit of vain dreams. Remember the dog's curly tail; every time it's straightened, it springs back. So it is with the world. Each person has his place in the plan. All that we are, as a society and as a planet, is based on the individual. How we manifest ourselves as a nation is based on our collective attitudes. If we are aghast at the lying and the cheating in government, we should be even more aghast that these attitudes spring from ourselves. When the individuals are multiplied to equal a society, the results are magnified proportionately. The world can change, but the tail can never be fully straightened; for life on this planet is not meant to be "all beauty and light." There certainly have been times when life was better, and certainly the future holds better times too, but it has not always been that way, nor should we expect it to always be so. After all, the world is a multitude of variables that produce, in their combination, ups and downs, never horizontal lines.

chapter two — Being Single, Being Married, and Being Divine

There are four basic stages in the life of a yogi: the brahmachari (student); the grihasta (householder); the vanaprasta (the couple without duties of the former); and the sannyasi (monk). The traditional way for the yoga aspirant was to start his tutelage under a master as a brahmachari, then get married and raise a family. And when his familial obligations were discharged, to gradually ease himself out of the world into the life of a monk. Life for the contemporary yogi is considerably different, not only in reference to this scheme, but also to the world around him. Now, among many schools of yoga, there are two separate and distinct life-styles: family life and the path of renunciation. This, however, does not negate the fact that there are other yoga life-styles practiced. In America, with its changing cultural patterns, there are a variety of unique life-styles; so consequently, yoga life-styles exhibit this variation too. In fact, there is probably a different life-style for each individual. If you do not fit into either category of renunciate, or family person, don't feel you are excluded from, or unfit for, the practices. Yoga is adaptable to any life-style and to any person. Yoga comes to any person who desires it, no matter what his station or circumstances are. The following is a brief discussion of the two major yoga life-styles.

Unmarried.

More people today are rejecting the notion that being a fulfilled person necessitates marrying and raising a family. Women especially are boldly striking out against this mold, finding life as a single person is not at all a lonely existence. An offshoot of this cultural change is that many people are realizing they're not suited for a married life, but rather, their swadharma is that of a single person. They view the role of a family person as a choice, not an obligation. There are, of course, many variations of unmarried living. People live with roommates, they live in a group, they live with their family, or they live by themselves. You may ask, "Am I single if I live with my boyfriend (or girlfriend)?" Technically, you are; in reality, you are not. This kind of arrangement is an informal marriage; you are sampling the married life without formally committing yourself to it.

Not all single people are suited to, nor want to live, the life of a renunciate, or monk. Single people have special life-styles of their own, which, under the impact of the yoga practices, has new dimensions added to it. Initially, a person may take yoga classes to improve his health or to learn the meditative techniques. Often, people go to these particular classes to meet others. If, however, you become involved in the practices in any way, something of your life will begin to change. You may have had a very active, whirlwind social life: parties, films, concerts, dining out, drinking. As interest in the practice continues, these particular aspects of your life begin to assume less importance. Relationships are struck up with other single people with similar interest, and occasionally small communes are formed. Among people sincerely interested in the practices, these habits and former aspects wither away on their own. No real, hard struggle is involved in overcoming the former habits. Within the short space of six months, I have seen people change from very worldly people to sincere spiritual aspirants. This kind of abrupt change does not necessarily occur in all cases. Remember the story about the damp logs; all possess aspects that take a long time to cure. Gradually infuse yoga into your life, and slowly your life will change. The most important thing a single person should remember is to establish the yoga practices within a supportive group. Then, after they are part of your life-style, move, if you desire, into a secluded, independent living arrangement. So, the progression can be: first, discard old habits; second, support the establishment of the practices; and third, set up a solitary, independent abode.

Married yogis.

The path of married people is different in kind from single people. While single people clear away that which is disturbing or superfluous, the married person engages in discovering and understanding the bond that exists between himself and his spouse. Usually, one person takes the initiative in instituting the relationship's direction. If it is a fairly new marriage, the spouse who takes the spear-heading role is sometimes viewed with concern by the other member, and a struggle for control ensues. If yoga happens to be the battleground, obviously, little spirituality will result in the relationship. If the couple gets beyond this critical phase, and discovers their shared bond, they can direct their attention to the task of uncovering the inner reality of the relationship. As they grow in this reality, they also discover themselves as individuals. It is in this discovery that they see their full potentiality to transcend the relationship. For a yogi, marriage may not be a forever thing. In order for this full flowering to come about, the initial support must be given. Most householders practice Karma yoga as their main discipline. The selfless path is the means by which the relationship flowers. It is this selflessness that overcomes the initial struggle for power. It is selflessness that binds the couple together, and it is selflessness that aids the individuals in rising above and beyond the relationship.

Great in their own way.

There is a wonderful story that illustrates how each of the aforementioned life-styles have their greatness. Once a great king asked all the wise men in his kingdom, which was the greater, the way of the householder, or that of the sannyasi? Many responded, but few gave him what he considered a satisfactory answer. When a few gave answers he agreed with, he asked for proofs. Unfortunately, they were unable to supply them. A young sannyasi came one day and responded to the king's question by saying that each is great in its own place. Again the king asked for proof, to which the sannyasi said, "If you will follow me into the forest, I will show you the proof you are looking for. So the king followed him out of his domain, into the kingdom of another. The princess of this kingdom was eagerly looking for a suitor, and as was the custom, she held audiences for all the eligible bachelors to be presented to her. Periodically, a general audience was held in which she perused the finest the kingdom had to offer. As the sannyasi and the king entered this assemblage, they espied a radiant young sannyasi on the outskirts of the crowd. Immediately when the princess saw him, she cried out, "That's the one," and threw a signifying garland around his neck. The young monk looked at the garland and disdainfully threw it away, saying, "I will not marry. I want none of this," and then calmly strode out into the forest. The princess was distraught, and she followed after him. The other sannyasi said to the king, "Let us follow them and see what happens." The young, pursued sannyasi, familiar with the paths of the forest, was soon able to lose the princess. She sat down on a rock and wept; not only had she lost the sannyasi, but also her way. The king and the other monk, finding her in this condition, told her not to weep, for they would help her out of the forest. But since it was getting dark, they decided to make camp for the night. A little bird family was perched high up in a tree above the wanderers. The father bird, seeing that the night was getting cold, said to his wife, "Dear, how cold it's getting. We should gather some firewood so that they'll be warm tonight." He quickly flew and got some twigs. He then went and retrieved a piece of burning twig from a nearby village and set the pile of twigs on fire. But as he looked down upon the company, he said to his wife, "Dear, what shall we do? There is nothing for these people to eat, and they must be hungry. As householders, it is our duty to feed anyone who visits our home. I will do what I can." At that moment, he flew into the fire and burned himself before anyone was able to save him. The wife looked down at the little bird and said, "There is still not enough for them to eat; one little bird is not sufficient." She too threw herself into the fire. The little baby birds, seeing the charred bodies of their mother and father, said, "Our parents

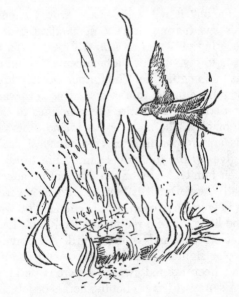

have done their best and still there is not enough; it is our duty to carry on their work." At which point, they too, flew to their deaths. The princess, the king, and the sannyasi, after seeing what they had done, could not bring themselves to eat the family of birds. In the morning, the king and the sannyasi showed the princess the way back to her home. As the two men traveled back to the king's providence, the sannyasi remarked, "You see, each is great in his own place. If you desire to live in the world, live like the birds, ready at any moment to sacrifice yourself for others. If you want to renounce the world, live like that young sannyasi who, faced with the riches of the kingdom, rejected them for his love of God. The life of a householder is one of sacrifice; the life of a sannyasi is one of renunciation. Each is divine."

Renunciation.

The life of a monk is not a life many would choose. Few are called to this swadharma; it is a demanding task, one which requires unceasing vigil and an iron will power. To renounce, in a yogic way, is to give up one's attachments; the relinquishing of which affects one's entire life. The former worldly life dies as the renunciate is reborn in the role of a sannyasi, or swami. Once he is reborn, he dedicates his entire life's energies to the unceasing service of humanity. The monk exists for no other reason. Thus the demands and responsibilities of a sannyasi are great. In a sense, they give up the individual family life to take on all humanity as their family. Many of you may not be interested in this particular path; however, it is beneficial to be aware of it, since all the paths in yoga have elements of renunciation within them.

What is the life-style of a renunciate like? Let's begin with the outside manifestations and work inward. A sannyasi wears orange. This color signifies that his desires and former mind impressions have been burned away, so there is nothing left of his former life. A sannyasi has no family, home, or job; he owns neither material possessions nor titles of rank. A sannyasi calls all countries, not one, his home. All families, not any one in particular, are his. He has no possessions, for he lives totally by the will of God. Whatever is given to him, he uses completely for selfless purposes. Renunciates are celibate. They refuse to be concerned with sex distinctions. They stand above the duality of man and woman. Rather, they seek to delve into the depths of their spirit. Only with this kind of understanding can a sannyasi be approached. Often, because some sannyasis are so jovial, people frequently discount the seriousness of their practices, and the discipline and preparation it involves. This particularly occurs in the West, where there is laxity in maintaining a respectful mien toward people. Many mistakes in protocol are obviously made. It is true that some Indian swamis find our naïvete refreshing; often, however, they may find it also crude. My teacher relates a funny story concerning his initial contact with Americans in this country. Once he was invited to a party, and after he arrived, a group of people quickly crowded around him, asking him "very serious questions" about yoga, while equally intensely blowing cigarette smoke in his face. We may have come a ways since then, though I am sure additional understanding of the life of a monk should increasingly be incorporated into the American consciousness.

Sanyas dharma.

Two important guiding principles in the monk's life are renunciation and dedication. These teachings give shape to the sannyasi's life. When we speak about renunciation, we are talking about severing oneself from that which is not spirit, severing identifications with the material world. Anything that acts to bind the sannyasi must be cut away. It is in this particular practice that the sannyasi uses the teaching of tapas, or austerity, to help burn away those impurities and attachments. It is also with a spirit of selfless dedication that the sannyasi speeds up the process of detachment. By offering himself up in service to the world, the monk is purified and cleansed of his worldliness and attachments. One of the most difficult practices that a sannyasi does is to live in the world while renouncing it. This kind of life does not suit anyone except the strongest. Romanticism is pushed aside and trampled on in this particular path. There is no place here for wild-eyed idealists. These sannyasi are powerfully practical people; they are mountains of strength, for they have endured all the tests that the world can throw at them. The yogi cloistered in a cave is an untested individual; he has gained nothing if he cannot cope with the challenges of the real world. And the real world exists everywhere, in the country as well as the city. There is no place where the world does not intrude. Peace should never be governed by environment. A sannyasi should be able to deal with any irritation, both large and small.

There was once a yogi who lived alone in a cave for many years, believing, as the years passed, that he had attained great yogic powers and lasting peace. One day he came down to the neighboring town and held satsang; all the people from the surrounding communities came to see him. Two young men had also heard of the great teacher and decided to attend. As they entered the house where the satsang was being held, the first one whispered to his friend, "Look, see how peaceful the yogi is." The second lad nodded quietly in response. He was intently watching the yogi. The two friends soon made their way closer to the swami, to ask him some important spiritual questions. After questioning the holy man about kundalini, meditation, and samadhi, the observant lad asked him if he smelled smoke. "What, my son?" replied the swami. "I don't understand." "Well, Swamiji, I really think I smell smoke." "Smoke? There is no smoke here," said the swami. He looked around to the other people. "Does anyone else smell smoke?" No one did. "See, there is no smoke." "Well," the young man insisted, "I know I smell smoke," and with that he began to sniff around the swami's chair. "Yes, yes, there is definitely smoke." The other young man thought his friend had gone completely crazy. "What are you doing?" he said. "There's no smoke here." "No, no, I really do smell smoke, and if you don't watch out, there'll soon be a great fire." "Stop it," said the swami. "There's no fire here; take your seat and be quiet." But the young man was not to be put off. "No, Swamiji, there's smoke here, and I can smell it." The swami was becoming quite agitated by now. "Won't you please take your seat? I believe we've all had enough of your antics. Now take your seat!" His voice was trembling in anger. Even with this rebuff, the lad persisted. "No, Swami, I can really smell the smoke even now. It's getting very strong, very, very strong." The swami got up and raised his hand to strike the lad. The youth backed away, saying, "There, there's the fire right now." "What are you talking about?" shouted the swami. "There is no fire," he yelled uncontrollably. "Yes there is, Swami," the boy uttered quietly. "I smelled the smoke, and now your anger is the fire. Everyone came here thinking that you were a peaceful man, but really, where is your peace, if you have a smoldering fire within? All your meditation in a cave has not doused that fire within."

The sannyasi must always be ready at any moment to face life's problems and vicissitudes, with equanimity and detachment. You may meet some young swamis or renunciates who have not been on the path that long and who appear very austere and serious, not at all like other jovial sannyasis you had met. This behavior should be understood in the proper light. At the onset of their practice, the sannyasi may feel his or her past life tugging at them. To overcome the old habits, the renunciate often has to keep close vigil on himself, in order to remain squarely on the path. Until he is internally established, this outward vigilance must be maintained. Part of the renunciate's path is celibacy. For the sannyasi, celibacy is a way of life, though certain of its aspects hold true for the other life-styles as well. Let us digress for a while and deal with the important and often misunderstood topic of yoga and sex.

Yoga and sex.

There are two frequently misunderstood concepts regarding yoga and sex. The first involves the beginning student, who feels that yoga looks negatively upon sex. The second takes the opposite stance and sees yoga and sex interconnected as a practice and a way of life. Both reliefs are incorrect and show a lack of understanding of the precepts of yoga. Yoga practices moderation in all things, and this is especially true with sex. Yoga believes that a powerful energy seed rests with the sperm which, if it is spilled frequently, depletes not only the man's physical energy, but his potential for spiritual energy as well. Many people find this a difficult pill to swallow. However, not very long ago, I was reading an article about a well-known rock star who, at the young age of twenty-nine, was taking vitamin-E supplements. It seems that his physical overindulgence was more than his body could handle. Yoga is not asking people to give up sex, but, again, the message is clear: as you become more involved in the yogic way of life, experiencing the deeper levels of awareness and peace, sex will become less important. To unite the self with the cosmic consciousness, and to go beyond the world of dualities, is the crux of yoga. In the sex act, though, there is a great trap that one can fall into, which is that the physical orgasm is akin to the cosmic one. Feeling this, people repeatedly emphasize the dualistic distinction between man and woman. They believe, to the contrary, that the physical orgasm is a means of rising above this distinction, which, in a small sense, is true. But the physical orgasm is nothing more than a mere substitute for the real ecstasy that man or woman can achieve. The real ecstasy happens with the severing of attachments and individuality. Real ecstasy changes the individual completely, and sexual ecstasy has never been known to change, or raise, him permanently upward. If changes do occur, they are usually of a more lascivious nature, as a result of their attachment to sex and sexuality. I realize that I am confronting a very thorny problem, which, in the midst of a sexual revolution, sounds like heresy. But yoga has never been part of a cultural revolution; rather, yoga has always done its own thing, maintaining a consistently high level of integrity, whether popular or not, for many thousands of years. Again, yoga is not against sex; it merely believes it to be a limited form of expression.

Moderation and celibacy, why people choose it.

There are people who choose celibacy (complete abstinence) or moderation (partial abstinence) as a way of life, who are not necessarily monks, nor planning to become monks. They have found this practice increases their peace and understanding. As celibates, they feel they are able to relate to people in a much clearer manner, without the discolorations of sexual overtones. It is difficult to relate to a person as a spiritual sister or brother if you are also relating to the person, whether subtly or grossly, in a sexual manner. If an individual desires to express spirit more than anything else, he chooses the moderate, or celibate, path, as a means to go beyond the dualistic extensions of man and woman. They are truly brother and sister in spirit. You may ask, "Is this a cop-out?" "Isn't the person just possibly running away from some underlying problem?" "Is he or she afraid of a relationship?" These are questions that are frequently put to yogis who maintain this way of life. The questions are fair; after all, it is quite possible that some individuals did use this way of life as a cop-out. However, the majority of people I know who have tried this path are men and women who have experienced relationships and sexually fulfilled lives. They chose this way because they have seen the inadequacy of a sexual life and the attachment and pain that sometimes come from this life. This applies to both single and married people. Many married couples seriously follow the moderate path. Family people especially are interested in practicing moderation simply because of the unreliability and sometimes dangerous results of current birth-control devices. Moderation and celibacy are the oldest, most natural, and safest birth-control devices man has at his constant disposal.

Celibacy and repression.

Due to the current freedom of sexual expression, and because this cultural revolution has come about as a reaction to the Victorian Age, people believe that celibacy is merely another form of sexual repression. Celibacy, if properly practiced, is control and not repression. Granted, some individuals are repressed, and they assume celibacy to further their suppressed personalities. Generally, these people have a difficult time of it; they often try escaping the world by moving away from people and the mainstream of life. Repressed celibacy is but a part of their personality. If you practice celibacy or moderation properly, you will find yourself to be a contented, open, responsive, and controlled individual. The will power derived out of the practice of celibacy is often needed in sustaining the practice itself. Some time ago, a teacher told me a story of his early days in an ashram under the tutelage of his master; and how constant vigil must be kept on this particular aspect of one's life. As he relates it, his teacher was going on a trip and entrusted the ashram's safety to the young disciple. As he was about to depart, he gave some final instructions to the student. "Now I want you to listen to me closely. Since this is an ashram, there should be no women visitors here while I'm away." The young swami nodded his understanding, and the teacher again looked at him deeply and said, "You must be careful of your own mind in these matters." The young swami again indicated he understood, and with that, the teacher turned and left. That night, there was a terrific rainstorm. From the front gate a woman's voice cried out, "Please let me in. I have nowhere to go and I need shelter for the night." "I'm sorry, madam," said the young disciple, "but I have been forbidden to let any women in while my master is gone." She again pleaded, "I was on my way to my mother's and I lost my way in this rainstorm. Please, Swamiji, let me in so that I can at least dry off; then I will be on my way. I promise not to disturb the routine of the ashram in any way." "But, madam," reiterated the swami, "I was forbidden to admit you or any woman." Insisting, the woman said, "I thought this was an ashram. Aren't you supposed to take care of all people? How can you turn me away in this driving rain?" The logic of the woman's argument caused a twinge of conscience. "Okay, you may come in, but you must stay locked up in a hut at the far end of the compound. No one

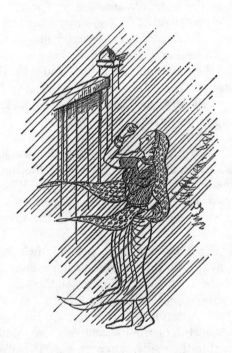

will be allowed to talk to you, and you will have to leave early tomorrow morning." The woman agreed to the conditions, and the door was opened. All covered up, she walked to the hut, thanked the young swami, and bolted the door behind her to lock herself in. The disciple then left for his own room. When he got there, he sat down to meditate. But as he meditated, the image of the woman kept coming back to his mind. He decided to go and check on her. Standing in the torrential downpour, he stood outside the hut. "Madam, are you okay?" "Yes, I am quite fine." "Do you have everything you need?" "Yes, don't worry about me, Swamiji, I'm fine." "Okay then, good night." "Good night, Swamiji." He went back to his room and since it was late, lay down to go to sleep. But he couldn't sleep; his thoughts kept returning to the woman, thinking about her face. Again he got up and went to the hut. "Madam, are you sure everything in your room is in proper order?" "Yes, everything is fine. There is no need to worry." "Nevertheless, I would like to take a look." "No," she said, "everything is really fine. Anyway, you instructed me to keep the door locked." "So I did." And with that he went back to his quarters. But still he could not sleep. An hour passed. Now he got up quite disturbed. Back at the hut, he knocked with considerable agitation at the door. "Madam, let me into your room. I must talk to you." "No," she cried out, "you cannot enter." "I don't care what you say, madam, I'm coming in." With quick movements, he climbed to the top of the hut and began ripping off the roofing with his bare hands. When he broke through the roof, he was startled and amazed to see his guru, alone, looking up at him from below, with the woman nowhere in sight.

The power of passion can drive men to such insanity. Men have been known to go to war over their passion; one immediately thinks of the Trojan War. Women, on the other hand, seem to have been able to control their passions to a certain degree. I am reminded of Aristophanes' comedy, *Lysistrata*, where the women en masse abstain from sexual relations until such time when the men stop their silly games of war. These women were essentially following the path of celibacy and moderation. People who practice this way, consciously have an idea and goal; they know exactly what they are doing. The reason behind the celibacy is one of direction and purpose, not of escape. The celibate and moderate person is interested in expanding, not contracting himself. Celibacy is at the core of renunciation. Repression is at the heart of attachment and bondage. To take full advantage of the practice, one must be mentally fit. If a person is practicing moderation as a means to escape, he will have little or no success in either endeavor. For when these individuals are exposed to the world and its higher equality, they will have no place to hide; and their repression will begin to crumble. Usually, such people try to compensate by running away from the stimulus, fearing that this is where the fault lies. But, of course, they take their problems with them, and there is no place in the world where temptation doesn't exist. As the young swami in the story found out, even an ashram is not safe from temptation.

Family life and celibacy. In family life, moderation is practiced with the goal of complete abstention in the future. Of course, what is moderate for one couple may not be for another. To practice strict moderation at the onset of the marriage can sometimes produce devastating results, particularly if one partner is more engaged in spiritual practice than the other. If yoga is to be incorporated into the family structure, then the whole family must participate in the practice, even if only in a small way. If the level, though, is made too high, then some of the members of the family will not desire to take part, and the joint spiritual feeling between the members will be lost. Some teachers recommend complete abstention for family members; some, once a month; and some put no limitations on the amount of times that the couple has sexual relations. I personally believe that the degree of moderation depends significantly on the couple's level of dedication to the practice. It is ludicrous to maintain a high level of moderation when both partners are not equally dedicated to it. Limiting sexuality does, however, establish the relationship on a higher spiritual basis. The great changes that occur within a couple, as their sexual life changes, does not affect the yogic couple who have been practicing moderation. It is easy to understand why divorces occur if they are based solely on sexual attraction. If the relationship is based on body and sex, then the interest will wear off quickly. If the relationship is based on spirit, there is no depth too deep for it to reach. So many young men and women are overly body conscious; they are no better than butchers looking for a good side of beef. This attitude which has trapped people into body identification permeates all levels of society. The institution of marriage and family has been seriously injured by it. So much attention has been placed on the orgasm and the multitudinous positions, one can only wonder where all of this will lead to.

Naturalness and celibacy. There is usually an initial awkward stage people go through in practicing moderation or celibacy. This should be expected and, if understood, can be dealt with in a very realistic and sound manner. Since sexual feelings are among the strangest emotions in the human psyche, one must understand that they will not dissipate quickly. When one takes the path of celibacy, dealing with one's sexual feelings is a long-term proposition. An active vigil should be maintained for the period of time that one is celibate. This does not mean locking oneself up in a closet; however, there are certain common-sense restraints that, when applied, will aid the person in his path of moderation. Naturally, finding a group of people who are of a like mind is very important. In fact, a path of moderation would be impossible to maintain in the company of immoderate individuals. Disturbing influences should be avoided at all costs. One should try to keep the environment around oneself as sattwic as possible, which means avoiding disturbing movies, books, parties, and even foods, which could make continuing on the path difficult. A person interested in pursuing this particular path should be cognizant of the restraints necessary to maintain it. This path obviously is not for everyone; there should be no guilt if you discover it is not for you. You can still benefit greatly from practicing the other disciplines. This now brings us back to the discussion about the renunciate's life-style.

Easing yourself into it.

To adequately determine whether or not you wish to live the life of a renunciate, you should test it out for a while. Experiment with various aspects of this life-style, by incorporating some of the practices into your present mode of living. Try the celibate path; live in a protected environment with friends who are following the path, or at a particular institution or monastery where it is practiced. Read books dealing with this life; spend time in seclusion. All these methods will assist the mind in deciding. Like celibacy, all individuals are not suited for this path. There is no higher or lower path. It is always better to do your own dharma, than someone else's. Once you have tried some of the aspects of this life, and you desire to get into it deeper, it is wise, at this point, to seek a teacher with whom you can ally yourself.

The needed protection of a renunciate.

From the outside, it may look as if a renunciate leads a prison existence. To the common-sense individual, one could not even conceive why someone would place himself in this kind of an environment. I remember, as a child, seeing an inexpensive paperback, entitled *Over the Convent Wall,* and thinking how terrible it must be to live in a convent. Only years later, after having met these religious people who lived "behind the walls," did I see and realize how truly peaceful and contented these individuals were. It is difficult to know (if one has not experienced it firsthand) the processes of a convent or any cloistered community. However, the walls are needed for the initial protection of the practitioners, so they may safely become established on the path. Certain influences of the world must be screened off. For instance, when you glue two pieces of wood together, you clamp them to aid the adhesion process. So it is with the monastic environment. It is like the clamp that aids in spiritual cohesion of the renunciate. The environment binds the individual with his practice, and thus, after awhile, they become wedded to those disciplines. Yogic monasteries are different from Western religious monasteries, most are not as secluded and withdrawn. They engage frequently in active social services, and often the communities around them are very much involved in their daily proceedings. In India, ashrams extend into the community, and the community extends into the ashram. So when I talk about the monastic model, it is good to keep this in mind.

Family life, problems and joys.

Family life is very much neglected in the descriptions of yogic life. The impression is given that the single person is the only one who can benefit from this life-style. Such is definitely not the case; yoga is perfectly suited for the family. A yogic family is one in which all of the members are dedicated to the same goal of self-realization. Life in a yogic family should be guided by a spirit of dedication and service. All members should participate in this spirit. This often does not occur, and family life, even spiritual family life, has it ups and downs. One reason for this is that parents, being what they are, cannot help but have expectations for their children; and children, being what they are, cannot help feeling the restraints of parental authority. Added to this is a prevalent tendency in our society for parents to be overly permissive with their children. As there are great joys in seeing one's children develop and grow up, so there also are great pains, for each successive developmental stage poses its own special problems. How a family deals with these successive stages depends greatly upon their own philosophy of living and, of course, their background. If the parents have been successful in transmitting spiritual values, and an essence of the spirit, then these particular developmental problems will not be given undue emphasis. However, if the parents lack stability in their own lives, these stages will be troublesome for them and, consequently, will ultimately pose problems for the child. Communicating the real sense of self is the highest duty that a parent has toward his children. We may give the child much in the way of material possessions, but if a sense of self is not communicated, we have given nothing.

The home as the temple. To provide an atmosphere in which spirit can manifest in the home, one must view the home as one's temple. It must be regarded as the central refuge, a sanctuary, from the world. If the spirit is not established in the home, then all members of the household will be looking for it on the outside. So how does one establish spirit in the home? First, the practices should be done in the home on a regular basis. Then, when the spirit manifests within you, all activities and members of the household will become spiritualized. Many people think that they have to set up certain rules and regulations within their home; actually, this is not necessary. If the initial task of discovering self is done, then all else will readily fall into place. For example, if a husband sees and experiences the yogic spirit, he will see it within his family and respond to it, thereby spiritualizing his family relationships. From this understanding, the entire household will know their responsibilities. Duties will be completed not as obligations to others, but rather as obligations to oneself.

Various spiritual practices can be performed as a family within the home. Doing this helps the spirit to manifest. Group chanting, or singing devotional songs, is an excellent activity in which both friends and relatives can join. These kinds of group sings can be followed up by simple and pertinent spiritual conversations, or readings of spiritual stories from the Bible and other spiritual books. These stories make very nice bedtime stories for children as well. Celebrating various religious holidays in the home can help manifest the spirituality of the family, when the entire family is involved in the preparations. It doesn't matter what religion you practice; pick those holidays you are especially devoted to. These things bind a family together and build a family tradition.

Doing spiritual practices in the open among your family is probably one of the most effective means of spreading knowledge about the practice and transmitting the spirit of yoga. Young children, naturally curious, are particularly open and receptive to the practices. Through their questions, they are essentially discovering the spiritual life for themselves. Take advantage of their curiosity by exposing them to a variety of spiritual activities. Older children may regard the change in the home environment with some suspicion. Try to introduce them to your practices by taking them with you when you visit your spiritual center or teacher. Let them attend a lecture or take a class by themselves. Do not force or coerce them, for such actions will only create dissention, and dissention will obliterate the spirit. Include the family in as many spiritual activities as possible. Invite spiritual people to your home. This not only fosters satsang, it also increases the spiritual vibration of your environment. If you can remain conscious that you are establishing a spiritual center within your home, then your home will serve the purpose for which it was intended.

Raising of children. Once the spirit is established in the home, there will be no child-raising problems; the children will raise themselves. A parent's main goal is to establish a sense of self in the child. This is done by transmitting to your child the essence of self that you have attained. You must be the best example. Parents are the child's first gurus. The yogic scriptures state that the child goes from the mother to the father to the guru and then to God. Parents have an important responsibility, for if the initial groundwork is not laid, the flower will bear no fruit. Educational philosophies and child-rearing practices mean absolutely nothing unless the sense of self is transmitted. One can give the best to a child, but if he has been starved of the spirit, he will wither from within. Conversely, one can give the worst to a child, but if he has been given spirit, he can overcome them all.

Viewing your mate as divine. The couple's spiritual model is exemplified in the relationship of Siva and Shakti. If the relationship is to be spiritual, then one must see one's mate as divine. A husband should worship his wife as a goddess, and a wife should worship her husband as a god. What does that actually mean? Does this mean that the wife should be a slave to the husband, and the husband a handmaiden to the wife? No, it certainly does not. It simply means that we look for the spirit within our mate and relate to it. In order to do that, though, one must first discover the spirit within oneself; because spirit can only relate to spirit. Some marriages are primarily based on body relations, while others are based on emotional needs. Others center on intellect, and still others are based on the spirit. Any marital relationship will simultaneously relate, to some degree, on all of those levels. A true and lasting relationship is principally based upon identifying with one another's spirit. Some people believe a marital relationship should be all spiritual. A relationship based solely on spirit, I honestly believe, is not a marital relationship and cannot last very long. There must be some modicum of physical, emotional, and intellectual satisfaction given, as well as spiritual. But even spiritual relationships, like other marriages, have had hard times and are not easily attained. Until this period of cultural revolution is over, secure marriages, whatever the basis, will be a rarity.

Dealing with a partner who isn't on your trip. Sometimes people get married who cannot agree on some basic aspects of their lives together. It is natural in the early stages of a union to find some disagreement or dissention. No groups, and relationships in this instance, are different; they all go through initial power and control phases. However, if one partner decides to follow the spiritual path and the other does not, the relationship not only has little chance of surviving but, even more importantly, has good chance of disturbing the minds of all concerned. It is therefore important to work the conflict out and expediently resolve it. Not everyone should be married, nor should everyone stay married; these are realities of life. To say this, I realize, does not lessen the difficulty in deciding whether or not to stay married. These decisions take time and obviously should be considered thoroughly. Sometimes, when an individual becomes involved in the yoga practices and the mate does not, he or she becomes very interested in casting off the spouse like an old shoe. This attitude shows a gross disrespect for another person. To force an individual into the spiritual life is completely at odds with the inherent message of yoga. One should be attracted by example, not by force. And, indeed, if one has become so blindly enamored with the practices, no matter how much you may tout the benefits, your spouse will never believe you; because he or she may feel that they are on the short end of the stick, that they have lost out to the yoga mistress.

Including spouses in the practice of yoga is the only way they can become familiar and at ease with the spiritual life. Resistance grows out of resentment at being left out. Indeed, you may try to include your mates in your yogic activities, but if they sense that there is an ulterior motive, that you are not doing it because you love them for who and what they are, they will balk. It is true that there is a certain level of adaption that one can make toward a mate without so diluting your own spiritual life. If your spouse, though, is adamant about your leaving the spiritual life to resume your former life, then there seems to be no real basis for continuing the relationship. Essentially, what you are trying to do is to gradually win your spouse over to your way of thinking. If you have tried all options and nothing has worked, then there may be no alternative but to go separate ways. However, as long as there is a glimmer of hope and a flicker of interest, fan it and see if, given some time, it will develop.

chapter three — Fast Ways, Slow Ways, One Way, and Your Way

In the first section we briefly mentioned the various schools of yoga and their respective claims. It is disheartening, and somewhat confusing, to see the various yoga practices competing with one another. Often, teachers of these various schools will meet on a public platform and proceed to argue and debate among themselves. This is sad to see, for it only serves to confuse the issue of the validity of the various paths. This book is not concerned with judgments; I do not propose to set myself up as a critic of yoga practices. For, in truth, I believe all practices are valid for some people. The number of people that the individual practices are valid for may vary, but all are worthwhile at least for some sector of the population. It is a shame that most yoga schools have not realized that each path is great in its own way. Oftentimes, in open discussion, they may admit this, but when a beginner or a new student comes, they engage in disparaging conversation about other paths. This not only creates ill feelings among the various schools, but gives the new student a very bad initial impression about the integrity of the yoga teachers. How easy it is to find fault if faults are being sought. Consequently, it is easy to hear gossip and pass rumors if one wishes to hear and believe such things to be true. The spirit of yoga is serious; fault-finding and gossipmongering have no place in it. If we wish to broaden the spiritual brotherhood, we must realize its presence among all the diverse yoga practices. This is no area for competition. Not out of competition but, rather, out of compatibility does a student attach himself or herself to a particular teacher and way. No amount of coercion can keep a student in a discipline he or she does not wish to belong to.

Evangelizing or active proselytizing are also not indigenous to the spirit of yoga. It is terrible to hear stories about traveling teachers who hypnotize and dupe unsuspecting students. It is sad that such things actually happen. An informed public is probably the only real solution to this problem. One should not condemn all of yoga because of charlatans; they abound in all professions and all sectors of society; yet still we respect the professions as a whole. Every year we hear about more quacks in medicine or accountants that have embezzled their clients' funds. Bogus teachers also have been heard of in the past and probably will be heard of again in the future. The way to spot bogus gurus is relatively easy. These teachers are mostly concerned with putting down other ways and touting *their* way as the fastest and the only way for God-realization.

Is there a fast way?

Naturally, new students are immediately interested in finding out whether the path they have chosen is a fast way. In America, where the culture often promotes quick and easy answers to all sorts of ills, it is not surprising that new aspirants bring this mental attitude to the yogic experience. Many teachers play up to this rather naïve attitude. This was especially prevalent years ago when yoga was primarily known as a physical culture. Teachers advertised it as a cure-all for every imaginable physical and mental pain. People with weight problems, arthritis, anxiety, and even more serious illnesses, came to these teachers looking to be told that yoga could cure them of a lifetime of bad living. Many of these people were taken very badly, and some are still being taken today. Yoga is more prevention than cure. There can be no quick and easy answers to a lifetime spent in bad habits. This is not to say that yoga cannot help, but it takes many years of proper yogic living to undo the problems of the past. As the attitude among new students became more serious and the desire for inner experience and knowledge more prevalent, students sought out teachers who could communicate this experience to them. They went to teachers who had developed powers, or siddhis, and, by means of thought or energy transference, gave the students some rudimentary experience. Since these beginning students were naïve, they took this experience as the bona fide spiritual one. They ceased their own inner searchings and looked for similar experiences in other forms. Interest in psychic phenomena developed. The occult, with its stress on manipulative power, attracted many students. People ran from one teacher to another, to experience the various tricks that these gurus could do. They would often meet in groups and talk about the experiences that they had; and although these people never developed occult powers themselves, most of them remained deeply attached to the occult perception of the world; spirit for them was something that could be manipulated at will.

Today students have gone beyond the occult powers, searching earnestly for teachers who can show them the proper practices for self-realization. Characteristically, they, like their forerunners, are looking for expeditious ways. This current attitude finds its roots in the psychedelic revolution of the 1960s. It was thought that psychedelics could, in effect, push you over to realization. People believed that with the help of American technology, "the grace of God," and Sandoz, a pill had been produced which could enable one to reach enlightenment instantly. Some experienced "enlightenment," but the vast majority did not. Their longing for enlightenment remained, and they now set out earnestly in search of teachers who could bring them that experience, quickly and easily.

Many wells, little water.

After psychedelics came the period of guru-hopping. Students eagerly sought a teacher they could study under. I do not belittle this quest, but with some people, the quest was nothing more than an exercise in futility. They searched with a preconceived ideal of a guru in their minds. Each teacher they encountered was compared and accepted or rejected according to likeness or dissimilarity to the mold. Naturally, reality rarely conforms to our mind's ideal; so, consequently, these people jumped from teacher to teacher, constantly searching, constantly dissatisfied; very much like young men searching for their dream girl. The romantic notions of what gurus and the yogic life are have become obstacles in the student's path of discovery. For example, *Siddhartha, The Autobiography of a Yogi* and *The Life of Milarepa* have sincerely affected many people spiritually. They start identifying with the main characters, searching for teachers with similar exemplary attributes. There was no way disappointment could be avoided. Romanticism is lovely, but in the day-to-day life of a yogi, it has hardly any place. When a beginning student attempts to find an unattainable teacher, he vainly moves from one practice to another, wasting valuable time and gaining little depth in his search for self. My teacher compares this behavior to a man who digs several shallow wells in search of water; but because he has dug many one- or two-foot wells, he will miss finding the water that is only ten feet underground. If, of course, he would have stayed in one place, he would have surely found it. In the quest to find the fast way, many have unwittingly chosen the slowest path possible. It is perfectly logical to try several ways before settling on any particular one. However, if the experimental period is inordinately prolonged, valuable time and energy are wasted. These people do not realize the extent their minds have been controlling them. Many times they are only carrying over habits that they have been living with their whole life; jumping from one thing to another; in and out of schools, jobs, relationships, and then, of course, the latest phase, yoga. When they announce to their friends that yoga, or this teacher, does not work, it comes as no shock because of their past behavior.

The fast way.

What we are saying here then is that the fastest way is the way that is right for you. To find that way and the proper teacher, you may first have to try several different paths. Try sticking to one path for a specified length of time, until you realize that either the path is comfortable, or the teacher is not suitable to your temperament or desired direction.

One discovers the fastest path when one is comfortable with the direction of the path. This does not mean life in general is comfortable, it simply means the student is in agreement with the practice. If this agreement is made, then the added ingredient for quickening one's development can be put in the recipe. This added ingredient is dedication. Once one has become convinced that the path that has been chosen is the proper one, the next and most logical step is to dedicate yourself to it. You might think that this is elementary, but it is not. There are many people who realize quite quickly what their path is but who have a very difficult time in getting down to the real work. They may fight with the teacher, or with the other students, questioning sharply the practices and the policies, sometimes running away altogether. Such was the case with the great Vivekananda, student of Paramahamsa Ramakrishna. Inwardly, Vivekananda knew that Ramakrishna was his teacher, but Vivekananda was young and rebellious, and only after his master died could he get serious about his practice. The result was that he flowered into the great and renowned yogi he is remembered as today. The fast way comes about when one takes full responsibility for one's life, looking to no one, nor anything, to bring that enlightenment. This does not mean that the student leaves the master, but in a sense, the master has said all that he can to the student, and the student moves on his own. The student knows what to do; he has listened to the guru's instructions and has internalized them. He then goes out and lives the message. Living the message with sincerity and dedication is the fast way and the fulfillment of the guru-disciple relationship.

Is there one true way?

Too often, teachers claim theirs is not only the fastest but also the only true way. This claim may be accompanied by a lot of double talk about the guru being in direct disciplic succession from a realized teacher or deity. Some teachers make grandiose statements to the effect that since they became enlightened at an early age, they are obviously blessed and chosen and therefore God's appointed guardian of the true way. Often, these claims are difficult to ignore, and among beginning students, many may ask the question, "How can I pass up a chance to be under the guidance of a perfect spiritual master?" This fundamentalist approach is making a direct appeal to one's insecurity; supplying a ready handle to grasp, to relieve the anxiety of not having a teacher, to be told what to do. Yoga is not for the man or woman who is too prone to anxiety, for in most cases, these people will attempt to reach out for something solid to alleviate that anxiety. Yoga is something very subtle, and unless the individual is solidly based in himself, he will not get through the trials and tribulations present on the yogic path. There is obviously no such thing as the one true path. Like the fast way, the true way is your own way, whatever it is. If you find you can achieve greatness by rolling down Main Street in a barrel, do it! The truth of each path is determined by each person who follows it. No one can state beforehand that something is right for you; that is your judgment alone. Blind faith and belief have very little to do with the yogic experience.

Belief should be tempered heavily with doubt. The two play

off each other, giving the individual a balanced perception. It is a fine line that the yogic practitioner walks, neither believing nor doubting in excess. To believe there is a true way removes doubt and takes away responsibility. No way can be true if it takes away individual responsibility. The real way is the path of truth. Individuals seeking the path of truth must be allowed to seek and find it themselves. That is the one true way, the path of understanding and enlightenment, which comes about through individual initiative. There is a little saying that I've seen recently which underscores this. It goes, "Give me a fish, and I eat for a day. Teach me to fish, and I eat for a lifetime." Give me enlightenment and I may be enlightened for a day. Teach me the way and I will be enlightened forever. But whether you teach me to fish or the way of enlightenment, I must do the work myself. This is a slow and steady way of development, but it is also a sure way.

Enlightenment does not come like a flash and go away. It is a steady progression, a natural evolution of consciousness. Enlightenment is the result of all the previous groundwork having been laid out beforehand. No teacher, great or small, can produce an enlightened person overnight. Nor can any obstacle, great or small, stop a well-prepared individual from reaching the final stage of enlightened consciousness. The true way is the path which leads you to a full expression of yourself.

When things don't happen.

There are three basic stages in a student's evolution which deal with the different levels of perception of his practice. In the first stage, there is an exhilarated feeling that you are working with the practice, and something is really happening. Often this is accompanied by a strong emotional tie to the teacher. In fact, you may even believe he is personally "pulling strings" on your behalf. In the second stage, nothing appears to be happening; you go from one day to another, plodding through your practices, feeling progress has virtually come to a standstill. Although the teacher is there, still doing the same things, nothing seems to be right. Whereas before you felt close to the teacher, now you often feel alienated and distant from him and the practices. This stage can last a long time and be quite frustrating. The third and final stage is one in which you have settled at a level of practice and can clearly see which particular areas of your study need work. There is an acceptance of yourself as an individual with limitations, but you also have the knowledge that there is great untapped potential. You work not so much with a goal, but with an understanding of every moment's importance. Many people have problems accepting the realities of the second level, especially after having passed through the euphoria of the first. Frequently, they are in an quandary as to what went wrong. The first level brings an intellectual and emotional, if not spiritual, understanding of the unlimited power to express spirit. This opens up an unbounded feeling of enthusiasm. But the wall of reality presents itself at the second level, and you find that indeed you are a limited being. The enthusiasm dissipates like smoke caught in a wind, quickly replaced by skepticism. If you are strong and desire to prevail and persevere, this skeptical phase will pass and balance out at the third level. The second stage is crucial; for many, disillusioned, leave the practice of yoga at this junction, to search for other endeavors to fill the emptiness they thought they had lost through yoga. However, sticking it out through the second stage will bring rewards in the third. There will be a union of such magnitude between your personality and psyche that neither words nor dreams could possibly conjure. It is now that your spiritual wings unfold in all their magnificent grandeur. But only through the pain of the second level can you reach the ecstasy of the third. In fact, a sure sign of your being on the right path is if, to some degree, it causes you pain. It is common for students to project inadequacies upon their teachers and leave during this difficult second period. This is unfortunate, for the student has probably already put in considerable time with the teacher. Occasionally, students are right in their choice to leave the teacher. The reason for leaving, however, should be because they doubt the practices, not the effectiveness of the teacher. Students, I fear, misconstrue the teacher's intent and, consequently, have notoriously incorrect perceptions of him or her.

How to find your own way.

Finding your own way does not suggest striking out on your own. Rather, it implies that your path be comfortable to you. In this way, you define what is important to you. Each person defines his own way by his particular tastes and temperament. Therefore, it is quite natural for students following the same teacher to all be slightly different. The master is influential in having the students evolve in an individualized way. This is contrary to the occasional misconception that the teacher attempts to mold students in his own image. A good teacher always guides the student in his or her own evolvement. A good teacher will show great forbearance and patience with the student's mistakes in order that he discover his way. Imagine the patience of a teacher who sees the proper way for a student and forbids himself the luxury of directing the wayward person. For the student must realize his own path; to be told what it is, does little good. The guru could tell, but if the student is not ready to listen, what is the use? So the student must make silly mistakes before he gets the message; and the teacher can merely point the way. The student must keep himself as open as possible; for in doing that, he is able to allow himself to change as he evolves. If clinging occurs while spiritual evolvement is taking place, great pain and confusion ensue. The easiest way is to keep loose and flow with whatever changes come about. If teacher and student are doing their parts, the student will manifest in his own individual way. What the student is actually doing in the world, and the actual finding of his way, may have little to do with each other. However, eventually, through the course of the evolution of his way, his situation in the world may well be affected. People may think "your path is set" and that you "know where you are and where you are going"; however, this characterization of your personality's worldly side has little to do with your spiritual evolution. One could be "set in his ways" and still be evolving spiritually. You could be going to the same job everyday, year after year, meeting the same people, and still be increasing in your awareness of the spiritual path. Spiritual seekers are, in a sense, members of a secret society, because the real spiritual work is done quietly, out of sight of most of the world's people. Only if you have eyes to see can you discern a spiritual person who goes about his worldly duties.

Evolution of spiritual consciousness is happening everywhere, and once you enter that awareness, you will discover people from all walks of life there. Everyone is following his or her own way, but all are brought together by one common denominator, the spiritual thread that is woven into the fabric of the world and the universe. As we become aware of our way and discover the thread running through our lives and all that we do, our paths become clear. This then is our connection to the brotherhood of seekers. Your own way has always been there, silently waiting to be discovered. Once you remove the final layers that veil you from it, you will experience a tremendous completeness and fulfillment that will immediately tell you that you have found the "Real Way."

chapter four — Busting Models and Busting Yourself

Living and growing in spiritual groups presents a problem in life-style identification. Some spiritual groups and people identify so strongly with their own group's "images" that they fail to realize and understand that spirit transcends these outer accouterments. This superrighteous morality of maintaining oneself, even one's spiritual self, above another is but another form of prejudice.

Life-style identification.

Oftentimes, spiritual students gather to validate their own beliefs. They carry this practice to such an extreme that reality is blocked and spiritual development is forfeited. As we noted before, social psychologists call such processes group-think. Essentially, members of the group reflect each other so completely that dissension or contrary opinions do not find expression. These groups of course answer some basic need for its members, i.e., support in establishing practices and developing life-styles. But in developing these aspects of an individual's spiritual life, group-think often runs rampant, especially in the early development of groups. Later on, after the group is established and the members have settled into their own lives, diversification and open criticism are permitted to exist unchallenged. Some groups take longer than others to reach this point, the group identity being so strong that members are wary of parting from it. Other than supplying support in the initial stages of establishing the practices, the group takes on the role of a crutch for the student when his spiritual "leg" needs mending. However, the trouble is that some people use it when there is no need. This obviously occurs more frequently with dependent individuals. If the individual discovers this tendency either in himself or in the whole group unit, his dissatisfaction with the situation may manifest itself in open group conflict, and the student is left in a very painful place. At this point, two things can happen: the student either leaves the group or develops an inner identification transcendent of the group's identity. A common tendency for students abandoning the group is to lay blame on it for their own problems. These people revert to their former identities, claiming them to be their real ones, frequently accusing the teacher of fostering a false identity on them. What has actually happened is that the students initially attach themselves to a spiritual identity; they gradually outgrow it and become disillusioned by this occurrence. They experience a great loss and spiritual void in their lives, and they return to the former life-styles that are well known and thus more real to them.

The trouble lies neither with the group nor the teacher but, rather, with the individual himself, who believes in a life-style identification and a false spiritual identity. Models are useful as long as they are considered just that, and not the real thing. Once you outgrow a model, you must move to a finer and subtler one; still careful not to misconstrue it for anything but what it is, a model.

Busting the spiritual model.

To bust the model, you must first know what it is you are destroying. This may be especially difficult and not particularly advisable to do in the beginning stages of one's spiritual practice. Certain realizations about the model must become apparent before you detach yourself from the world. It is a transition life-style that directs and leads you to your real one. If you understand that the real spiritual life-style for yourself is not something that you can quickly pick up and put on like a coat, then you will have taken the first step toward busting whatever model you live by. We all live by models; sometimes one, sometimes many, sometimes spiritual, sometimes not. The goal of yoga is the disintegration of these models, for until these models are removed, the real spiritual life cannot manifest itself. Many people don, and attach themselves to, the renunciate's model in their zealousness to manifest their inner life. Their attachment is so strong that they eventually become more possessive about the model than they were about their former lives. This is ludicrous at best. Others swing like pendulums, alternating from one spiritual life-style to another, from rigorous disciplines to lax ones. They seem to live several lifetimes in a brief interval of time. If a psychologist were to look at them, they might think that they were schizophrenic. But no matter how absurd, it is all part of a natural process of an individual ridding himself of models. Sometimes the student is serious and conscientious about his practice, other times jovial and nonplused. Viewing these people from the outside, they give the appearance of drifting and flowing with the spiritual group. If you know such people, or are one yourself, there is no reason to fear these occurrences; for the process is natural and eventually will lead you to the discovery of your own spiritual life-style.

Supportive groups.

There are many varieties of spiritual groups; some are very open and loose, while others are very closed and strict. All spiritual groups support the direction of their own particular models. As such, groups, whether spiritual or not, provide identities for their members. But often, people expend tremendous time and energy with their one particular spiritual group, thereby relying heavily on that group's model. This results in a sharp decrease in activities outside the realm of the spiritual group. For friends and relatives of a student in a group, this sharp drop in outer activity can be alarming. It is a typical response of any person who wants to immerse himself in the spiritual life, and unless the individual is deeply disturbed, it should be viewed as temporary. Sometimes this period of reclusiveness will last for months, other times it lasts for years. But almost always, all students eventually shed the protective shield the group has given them and establish, to some degree, a life of their own. A well-balanced supportive group will make sure that the individual deals with the outside world, to some extent, even in the midst of very serious involvement with the group. Wanting to set up your "own life" too early can be detrimental to proper spiritual evolvement. This often happens when especially "perceptive" students see faults in the spiritual model and feel that, by setting up their own life, they might transcend the group.

The model may present itself quite clearly to you, thus enabling you to discern which parts of it are applicable to your situation and needs. In fact, you may feel that other people (who have identified with it more closely than you) are excessive in their identification with the model. But the question is, How much commitment does the model warrant to be effective? To transcend the spiritual model one must be totally committed to the group. To stand on the outside and criticize is a meaningless endeavor. True, honest and helpful criticism can only come from the person who knows the internal mechanisms, that is, from a participant, not an observer.

In America, and especially now in the 1970s, there is a great deal of mistrust directed toward organizations and groups. The feeling that the way of the rugged individualist is best still prevails. Groups and organizations are looked upon as dehumanizing and, potentially, even detrimental to the individual as well as to society. That is why many people refuse to join any spiritual group and look, from the outside, with disdain on the activities that take place. They belong to what I call the eclectic spiritual group, a very supportive model which, like other groups, has deep roots of identification. These individuals feel all teachers are beautiful; all ways are real; and consequently practice several bits and pieces from a variety of spiritual disciplines. This patchwork thinking may well be caused by a fear of the group as a manipulative agent that demands commitment as it strips away their freedom. Such thought processes constitute a very deep attachment which, unless looked into with great care, can become very destructive. Therefore, what I have been saying about supportive groups holds true as well for this particular group. The difference lies in that the latter group will find greater difficulty in transcending its model because its "members" believe they have already transcended it. To be a spiritual dilettante is possibly the most convoluted spiritual life-style identification one can have. Within the dilettante supportive group, individuals move randomly from one thing to another, never really staying at anything long enough to see its limitations and/or possibilities. It is like trying to hit a moving target.

Transcending the supportive group.

Since we've discounted leaving the group as the answer to finding one's life-style (though we also recognize that the vicissitudes of the supportive group cannot be stood forever), the solution is to stay as long as possible with the group and transcend its model. This is accomplished by involving yourself fully in the group life; experiencing the vagaries of the group's development, while at the same time, internalizing the group's model as your own. You must play the role and live the part convincingly, while retaining the belief and knowledge that the group's life is not your real life.

If this process is done completely, then the individual should never feel the need to physically leave the group of his or her own volition. But sometimes circumstances evolve and inner voices are heard which seem to point toward an imminent departure. How can we discern if they are real and what our actions should be? How can we know if our disagreements with the group come from our selfishness or from out of natural evolutionary growths?

First, before answering these questions, determine how deep the disagreement is and see whether you agree more than disagree with the group on any number of areas. If you are predominantly in agreement, there is a good basis for the relationship to continue and for you to cope with what probably is some small selfishness on your part. If the reverse is true, you may have to leave and search elsewhere for a supportive group that offers more areas of interest in common. But if after having spent many years with a group, you decide there is no common interest, I strongly recommend that you re-evaluate your perceptions and think over your reasons for leaving. Leaving should not be sudden for those with many years of involvement. I realize, though, that mounting disagreements over a long period of time force people to make what looks like a sudden decision. But if there are still large areas of agreement, you should bear up with the mind's disagreement and view it as a personal opinion, something which you would do otherwise if you had the power. But like the proverbial man on the street who talks about how he would run the government better, realize that you are not in charge and that, for a while, the powers that be have decided you must learn to follow precepts contrary to your own. The humility that accompanies such a practice will provide you with a properly balanced perspective on your own preciously held ideas. In this way you will be able to use the supportive group and its seemingly negative influences to your positive benefit. If you trust and love the members of the group, you will allow them to bust your personal model with the weight of the group model. Your personal opinions will not necessarily disappear. They'll remain; you will simply not be as attached to them as you were before. Having once reached beyond your own model, you will soon attempt transcending the group's. Holding one's own opinions and self-image are two important reasons for difficulty arising between the group and the individual member.

There are some people who hold no individual model and, because of certain pathological conditions, attach themselves to a group in order to gain self-identity. These individuals never transcend the group model, and unless the teacher forces them toward some deep re-evaluation, they spend their life mouthing spiritual platitudes. This may assist them in future lifetimes, but as to the present one, it is undisturbed and to a large extent, unfulfilled.

chapter five – The Simple Life for Hard Times

Hard times.

There is no doubt that there are difficult times ahead for the people in this country. The high cost of living and unemployment are forcing many people to re-evaluate their life-styles and seriously cut back on acquiring material possessions they once thought necessary. Shortages of natural resources and the high cost of manufacture have made formerly obtainable material objects unfeasible. Cars are being made smaller and more economical, and homes are being heated with less fuel. The country as a whole is becoming economy conscious. These have become desperate times for some people and caused them, in some instances, to take their lives, rather than face the challenge of changing them. Yoga views poverty from two perspectives. The first kind of poverty is forced poverty; that which a person or a family finds themselves in because of seemingly uncontrollable circumstances. The second kind is that which is embraced voluntarily. This does not mean solely the poverty of a renunciate but, more or less, living frugally because situations warrant it. For example, students often embrace poverty because they must spend the majority of their money on books and tuition. They know that it is a temporary circumstance and one with which they do not identify. The major characteristic of the second type of poverty is that the individuals do not feel they are poor, even though they are in the midst of poverty.

The first type of poverty yoga regards as a product of karma and, as such, sees the full responsibility for being in the culture of poverty resting on the individual. This does not mean to say that yoga blames the victim of the circumstance of poverty, but it does regard the poverty-stricken individuals and family as people who have the ability to change their own destiny. Social service agencies included, yoga feels that the individual, first and foremost, has the ability to wipe out and abolish poverty. Now, before anyone becomes too excited about what may seem to be a reactionary stance, let me further add that yoga realizes that some people have been victimized, and exploited, and, because of this, have found themselves in a state of poverty. Yoga realizes, too, that poverty cannot be completely eradicated from the world. There will always be some people poorer than others. There will always be some people exploiting other people less fortunate than themselves. And because of that, there will always be the state of poverty to work out those things in man's karma that only the particular circumstance of poverty can do. If one believes in the laws of karma and reincarnation, then one can see that the karma of being born into a culture of poverty may be an apt lesson for former unconsciously exploitive individuals. If one can learn the lessons of spirit in a poverty culture, then one can learn it anywhere. Spiritual evolution happens quite freely among the poor. People have risen above their level of poverty, not only by fame and monetary attainment, but by manifesting and expressing their spirit, thus transcending the level of their socioeconomic state.

Atheists probe at man's condition: "If God exists, why is there so much suffering and need?" This is an important question and has no simple answer. We cannot dismiss millions of people by simply saying that it is their karma. However, we must also understand that their karma placed them there, thus we should be compassionate and understanding of their plight and do whatever we can to alleviate their suffering. We cannot undo the situation, but we can lessen the burden. And perhaps in showing compassion toward others' sufferings, we can discern some of God's plan. For if there was no suffering in this world, would we care to ask the question, "Isn't there something more than this?" Perhaps those who are most rudely awakened are those who are slumbering the deepest. By understanding people and showing compassion, meaning can be brought into chaotic experiences, and a small light can be lit to illuminate the darkness.

The second type of poverty is one which is taken upon oneself for a specific reason or goal. This is the spiritual life-style that I would like to talk about, although it has manifestations, as I have explained above, in other more worldly contexts.

Material fasting.

As we fast to eliminate accumulated toxins from the body, so we embrace a simple life-style to eliminate accumulated attachments to unnecessary possessions. We may all be familiar with Christ's description of the spiritual destiny of a rich man which exemplifies this belief. Jesus said that a rich man has as much chance of getting into heaven as a camel has of getting through the eye of a needle. Perhaps this spiritual instruction was originally used as a rationale for accepting and embracing spiritual poverty in the monastic tradition. However, I believe the import of the statement is equally applicable to twentieth-century life. It is not that a rich man cannot enter heaven; it is that any man weighed down by his identification with his material possessions can never soar heavenward; and heavenward, for the yogi, is the inner state of bliss. Just as one wants to achieve a purified body and mind through fasting, so it is that one wants to achieve a state of balanced mental attitude by the elimination of burdensome material possessions. Please do not think that I am advocating throwing away everything that you own. I am talking about slimming down to a reasonable life-style, and not some ascetic ideal. Asceticism, as I have indicated before, can sometimes be the heaviest mental attachment an individual can have.

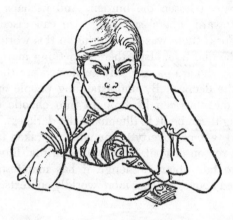

Benefits of material fasting.   Immediate benefits can be attained by making one's life-style economically based. Today, not only is everybody on a food diet but a money diet as well, desperately trying to spend less and save more. Money should be looked upon as concretized energy. We are reimbursed monetarily for energy used in the performance of our jobs. We work for the money, but it represents the energy we expended. We naturally want to conserve as much energy as possible; not expend it on useless items or activities. To do that would be to fritter away our preciously spent energies. So conservation of energy is a major benefit one gets from eliminating wasteful living habits. An additional benefit is a relaxed and peaceful mind. Being freed from worry about possessions naturally produces this state. Relinquishing these possessions in the beginning can be very painful. Sometimes, if done too quickly, a reaction to the practice develops. You start to wonder why you gave away something and how you will ever live without it. However, if you persevere through this period, a lighter quality will enter your life, and you will realize these objects were not really necessary. In the case of objects like TV and entertainment paraphernalia, if these are given up for whatever reason, one develops other means for entertaining oneself. We all decry the dependency that we have on these objects, along with the destruction of interpersonal communication and relationships that have evolved because of that dependency. It is not that these material possessions are of themselves bad; it is just that we overuse them and, consequently, become dependent upon them and lose the sense of naturalness that should be our life.

We have pyramided ourselves on a culture dependent upon technological advancements and the conspicuous consumption of them. People drive rather than walk to the neighborhood store. We use calculators rather than our heads to do simple arithmetic. Yes, we should use these conveniences, but should we overuse them beyond necessity? To pursue a spiritual existence, we must resist such trends and move toward a life of self-reliance. Doing without these conveniences, and making do with what one has, develops a sense of self if one is inclined to see it that way. Some years ago, there was a black-out that affected almost the entire East Coast of the United States. All electricity was out; people were caught at the five o'clock rush hour in such undesirable places as elevators and subways. They were forced to break through the impersonality of their existences and relate to each other on a human-to-human basis. Families rediscovered themselves. People had to rely on each other, and they found it to be a very rewarding experience.

I have been in situations where I have not had much in the way of material things, nor have the people around me. Although our condition didn't eliminate fighting and bickering, we are aware today, some years later, that because of the hard times we went through together, we are all very close in a special way. We laugh and joke about it now, but we realize that we were thrown back on ourselves because of the difficult situation, and we all tried to make the best we could out of our lives. Most of us were from middle-class families, and because we had chosen to live in the country, we had accepted our voluntary poverty as a matter of course.

Some examples of the simple life.

There have been people throughout history who have chosen to devote their lives to others, and not for the accumulation of material possessions. Albert Schweitzer was such a man. He devoted his life to the service of others. As he administered to the medical needs of the people of Gabon, he found little inner desire for material possessions or personal luxuries.

Mahatma Ghandi, with no more personal possessions than his sandals, loincloth, and glasses, changed the course of history for India and the entire world. Prior to involving himself in India's struggle for independence, he lived a relatively comfortable householding existence, having a fairly successful law practice. His complete dedication to the way of ahimsa and passive resistance broke British rule in India. When he traveled from one place to another, he didn't carry several valises with him. His personal possessions consisted of what he had on his back. When the police would come to arrest him, he would merely grab his glasses and put on his sandals and leave. He was not necessarily opposed to people having possessions; he was simply a man completely dedicated to his cause.

The lives of Schweitzer and Ghandi were extremely spartan but only because they led dedicated, spiritual lives of service, which far surpassed their needs for the trappings of the material world. Therein lies the key message to the simple life. It is not that you have to give away anything; it is more that as you dedicate yourself more fully, those things which you once considered important will no longer mean anything to you.

There are many spiritual people to pattern our lives after. St. Francis of Assisi, Thoreau, and John Muir also exemplify the principle of living a simple, spiritual existence. Their lives became simple merely from the fact of the way they lived. Questing, as they all did, for the spirit was their consuming passion, and they would not waste the time or energy in seeking the small and transitory pleasures of the world.

Self-sufficiency and co-operatives.

Now, because more and more people want to lead a self-sufficient life, the need has arisen for co-operatives, in order to save as much money as possible and to spend less time working to acquire the essentials of life. Food co-operatives have been established for some time. They are usually organized by a group of friends or neighbors who buy food wholesale and share the savings among the members. Though discounts can be considerable, there is, nevertheless, a lot of co-ordination involved in storing and distributing the food. However, many participants consider the time and energy put into the project well spent. A new co-operative was formed in the East which buys and distributes a variety of manufactured goods. They have even put out a catalogue for nationwide distribution. These co-operatives are basically geared for people who desire to be self-sufficient. Leading a simple life, though, should not mean leading a life of dependency. One should not have to go on welfare in order to become "independent," for a life on public assistance is nothing but a life of real dependency. The reason people choose self-sufficient living is so they can be free of depending upon other people. Dependency disturbs the mind, and one of the most disturbing aspects of American life is public assistance. Long lines and intimidating and embarrassing questions are all designed to compel the individual to remove himself from the public-assistance roles. A simple life should be lived self-sufficiently. To do this, your life-style must change. In no way, however, am I advocating a life of poverty for everyone. I believe in having wonderful and beautiful material goods, but they should not have you.

If, as part of your spiritual evolution, you desire to change your life-style and throw away some of the accouterments of a past one, then it is important to explore the possibilities of a simple existence. Co-operation with other people and maintaining a sense of self-sufficiency are integral aspects of this life-style that should be quickly developed. Search out bargains; visit thrift shops; swap unused clothing. Many avid thrift-shop hunters have furnished their homes beautifully from these stores. With creative imaginations and trial and error, it can be done. Food costs can be cut considerably if you grow your own vegetables, and this is applicable to both country and city living. A plot of land can be a window box as well as a "back acre." In other words, if you wish to survive, you learn how to do it.

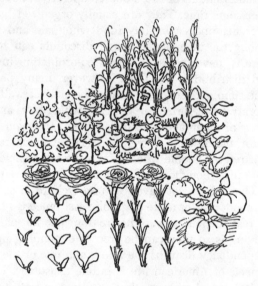

chapter six – Perfection in Action

The meditative attitude.

In talking about yoga and life-style, it is important to note that yoga cannot be practiced just for a few moments in the morning and then forgotten about until one decides to pick it up again. In order for yoga to be really effective, it must be practiced every moment of every day. The meditative attitude must be developed in everything that you do. Every action must be a meditation. Yoga integrates the inner practices with the life-style. The inner practices help one purify and concentrate on the inner spirit. But the realized spirit is manifested in the perfection of one's every action. The Bhagavad Gita succinctly says, "Perfection in action is yoga." Thus, everything you do, speak, and think is oriented toward purity, concentration, and absorption. One's actions must begin by being pure, and motivations must be selfless. This done, one can concentrate on the action, become absorbed by it, and eventually be at one with it. This is a perfect moment, what humanistic psychologists call a peak experience.

It happens to many people of diverse interests. Sports stars relate losing themselves in the game as their concentration becomes one-pointed. Actors, after months of rehearsing, become immersed in, and absorbed by, their roles. This is the essence of the Stanislavski method of acting. Great musicians experience this unique oneness; as they play, they give themselves totally to the music and let it flow through them. Perfection in action is at the core of the yoga teachings. Yoga is nothing more than the student's attempt at stringing together as many peak experiences as possible. Rigid concentration is not necessary for these types of experiences to occur; rather, concentration should be an easy and natural action of the mind; nothing is forced. By meditating, you will acquire the model for concentration that is applicable to many situations.

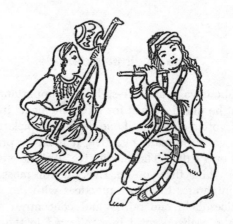

Concentration on the physical action.

When we sit and meditate, we constantly bring our roving mind back to the mental idea, image, repetition, that we have placed there for that purpose. So it is with concentration on physical action. We must constantly bring our minds back to the task at hand. This seems to be simple enough, for, in reality, we know that if we want to get something done, that is what we must do. But actually, most people only put half of their mind on the physical action they do, and half of it is wandering on some internal dialogue. The effort of a student should be on stopping the internal dialogue and placing the full concentration on whatever one does on the physical plane.

A secretary of Mahatma Ghandi was once asked what made Ghandi different from other people. The man responded, "Most people think one thing, say another, and do a third. Mahatmaji thinks, says, and does one and the same thing." This is the ideal for the person practicing meditation in action. Often in performing any chore, we break for respites to let our mind wander from the task. It seems that the mind needs this kind of flight of fancy in order to continue the task ahead.

This happens because we are concentrating improperly, and the only way the mind can rest is by drifting amorphously from focus. However, if you are relaxed and at ease in your work, the desire for rest periods is lessened substantially. Apropos of this is Ghandi's response to a journalist's query, "Why don't you ever take a vacation?" "But," he responded, quite surprised by the question, "I am on vacation!"

In the workaday world, so many people look forward to their vacations as an absolute necessity because the work is regarded in the light of being an obligatory duty; not something to focus one's concentration on. What one does is not as important as how one does it. It is sad that we put so much importance on status and class, for this obliterates the real functions of having work. They are, in their essential sense, objects to concentrate one's attention upon. If one looks at work, and all physical actions, in this light, then everything becomes a joy, because it becomes an opportunity to practice. Thus when mistakes are made, we can look at them as opportunities for improvement rather than areas of failure. A true yogi thanks the person who has pointed out a mistake; he never resents him. Perfection in action is something that should extend not only on the physical realm, but on the verbal and mental realms as well. In your daily interactions with people, you should strive to make those relationships as perfect as possible, reflecting deeply the purity of your motives and the perfectness of your action.

When to, and when not to.

All that I've said up to this point should not be construed to mean that yogis remain passively by, and do not enter, the mainstream of life. A yogi, like anyone else, can raise his voice in protest to something he feels is inappropriate. What we are saying is that meditation in action is knowing when to say what. It is essential to know when to keep quiet and hold back and when to go ahead and speak up. When one has become purified, one begins to experience that understanding. The divine spirit, moving through the individual, assists the student in deciding what is right to do. Without this level of purified thought, one's decision-making processes are apt to be weak and vascillatory.

Often, a beginning student of yoga will vascillate from one decision or option to another, desperately wanting to do the right thing, while knowing that to "desperately want to do the right thing" is a motivation of self-interest and therefore not the best route to take. Consequently, discerning the best motive and action for a situation can be a very trying task for the yoga student. For very often, one thinks that one is doing something in an unselfish manner, and it is only later that one discovers a whole new side of selfishness that was, in a sense, so subtle as not to be detected. That is why meditation in action can be a very helpful exercise in self-discovery, for only in the world are the great lessons of self learned. Only when one is on the firing line of life does one come face to face with oneself. Thus it is important that you reflect before you act and reflect after the reaction is received.

Touching the world lightly.

Since most yogis exist in the everyday world, they must master the art of touching the world lightly; moderation in everything, extremism in nothing. So many of us are used to overindulging ourselves by doing and saying more than is necessary. If one maintains the proper attitude, there is no need to speak or act excessively or elaborately. You should give of yourself, but leave the ego out of it. When one learns this beautiful practice, it is like walking on the beach without leaving footprints. Everything and everyone around you will be affected by your presence, for you will leave an indelible mark on their souls. This is the only print that a true yogi leaves when he departs.

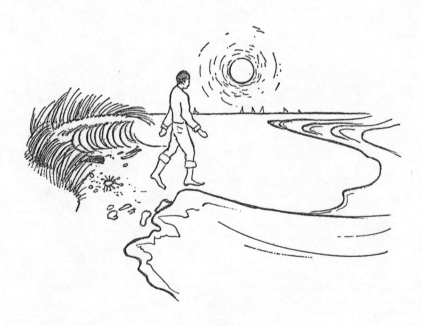

part four

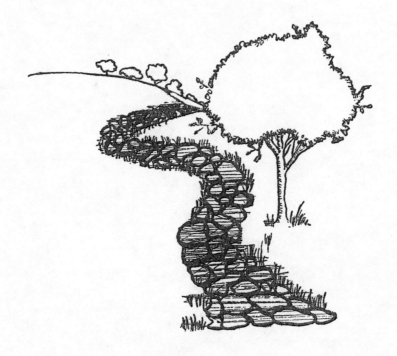

the
wedded way

chapter one — Yogis Speak

Introduction

We have now come to the part in this book where I must "put it all together." That is why I have called this part "The Wedded Way." For in order to have a truly effective yoga, one that is balanced, it must be integrated. Not only must the internal practices be integrated, but the practices themselves must also be integrated into life. Thus there is a double wedding, so to speak, among the practices and to life. That is what is called *Integral Yoga*, and that is why yoga is properly known not as a philosophy, or as a set of practices, but as a way of life.

Integral yoga.

The practices. Integrating the practices of hatha, raja, japa, bhakti, karma, and jnana yoga is designed to develop all aspects of the spiritual individual. Hatha develops the physical, raja and japa the contemplative, bhakti the emotional, karma the dynamic, and jnana the intellectual. Integral yoga believes in developing all sides of the individual to bring about a harmonious and balanced personality. If one of the disciplines are practiced to the exclusion of the others, oftentimes these neglected areas of the person become obstacles. A person who only meditates is often devoid of emotion, as an exclusive karma yogi can lack the calm center of the raja yogi. All disciplines should be practiced for maximum development on the path. Naturally, not all the disciplines will be practiced equally, but all should be practiced according to the capacity and the temperament of the aspirant. If this is done properly, all the elements of the aspirant will be healthy and in perfect harmony with each other. Then the individual can use these elements to transcend his individual nature and experience the divine.

The life. As the aspirant becomes purified and more one-pointed from the practices, he notices that his life is changing; that it has taken on a sense of purpose and direction. This is the Integrated Life, a life of spiritual dedication. It is a life where one sees whatever one is doing as divine intervention. The Divine Plan manifests in the aspirants' daily activities, no matter what they are. Butcher, baker, candlestick maker can all see themselves as part of the Divine workings, if they have the proper attitude. There is not one way, nor one model, to show as the proper way for spirit to manifest. For each person, it will be different. There are no robots in yoga; out of God we were all created differently, and we must live our lives in the way that was meant for us.

Some examples of the integrated life. Below are several interviews with followers of the integral yoga path. They were recorded in and around the Satchidananda Ashram in Pomfret Center, Connecticut. Their experiences on the path vary from many years to just a few. Some are sannyasis, some are single people, and other are householders. Many work for the ashram; some have jobs in the community. Some of the householders live in the ashram, and some live around it. Included is an interview with the most experienced member of the ashram, my guru, Sri Swami Satchidananda. It is Gurudev's interview which starts this section, and I feel it gives a wonderful overview and perspective to the succeeding comments.

The master's voice, an overview.

Gurudev Sri Swami Satchidananda, Founder-Director Integral Yoga Institutes, Satchidananda Ashram.

The entire practice is aimed at keeping the whole person clean and fit. All the practices, whether it is hatha yoga, bhakti yoga, karma yoga, or raja yoga, have as their aim keeping oneself clean. For example, breathing is a kind of cleaning, while at the same time it gives you vitality, making you healthier. First clean it, make it healthy, and then have control over it; that is the aim of every practice. Take bhakti yoga for example. It deals with the emotional side; the aim being to clean the mind and make it more interested in something higher, which we call God, instead of running here and there with thoughts of worldly things. Then you can offer everything to God; that means you are cleaning the mind. Instead of offering everything to worldly things like your nightclub money and your gambling debts, in bhakti yoga you still use the same money but you buy nice food, some beautiful flowers, and set up an altar. Both involve an expense, but here you are doing it in the name of God. Then when you use the food, flowers, and the altar in the form of puja, you are bringing the mind closer and more one-pointed. In that way you get the mind to stop going out to satisfy the senses. Thus by giving the mind to that which is simple, that which is God, and offering all the desires to God, you purge out all the undesirable things. So you see, in concentrated puja and service, the mind becomes more one-pointed, and at a certain point in the future, it becomes very calm. The same thing occurs in raja yoga. First we purify the mind with practices like pratyahara, yama, and niyama, purging out all undesirable influences. Then through meditation, we make the mind one-pointed. Karma yoga also does the same thing. Instead of going and doing everything just to satisfy your own ego, you do it in the name of others, to benefit others. It's a sort of dedication. That spirit of dedication itself makes the mind more peaceful, because anything that is done with a selfish motive disturbs the mind. If you get your desires fulfilled, you are excited; if you don't, you are depressed. Either way it disturbs the mind. But if you do an action with a selfless spirit, you don't worry about the loss or profit, you just do it, and have the satisfaction inside that the job was done well. There is no personal loss involved, nor personal profit.

So all these things are indirectly and directly helping a person raise above the individual self, a self-denial you might say. You deny the self to accept the higher self. That is what is called practice. When the mind gains control and it's healthy, your entire life is changed; then the entire life becomes the yoga practices. Whatever you do is the practice. Otherwise, if you simply do your puja, hatha yoga, and stop there, and don't apply that kind of attitude in your daily life, it's something like you earn a lot of money, put it in a safe, lock it up, and don't use it. What's the use of getting that money then? The fruit of those practices should bring certain good results in your daily life. Don't you agree with me? When your life becomes the practice, then the need to do the formal practices isn't very necessary. This is because everything you are doing becomes a form of practice. But still you might be doing something because to stop doing it is like stopping to wind the clock. It runs, and slowly it gets looser; the mind and body are like that. But if you have really established the spirit in the mind and body from the beginning stage, you will need less practice. That's what Ramakrishna Paramahamsa said; as long as the vessel is brass or copper, it can get tarnished quickly, so you have to keep on cleaning it at least once a day or once a month; but if you make it a golden vessel, then there is less opportunity for it to get tarnished, but it still needs to be cleaned. There is a certain stage where you just clean it while working. You don't have to do something different; it's sort of like an automatic watch, you have no need to wind it. Every time you move the hand, it winds automatically. So it is with yourself, you wind it up; you don't need to go and do something especially in the name of puja, everything becomes a puja for you. Even your ordinary breathing becomes a deep breath, and you don't need to sit and do special pranayama; the breath itself becomes pranayama. You won't have shallow breathing.

Proper diet will take good care of the body. Since the body is always relaxed, you don't get stiff, so you don't have the need to do Hatha yoga. Hatha yoga eliminates the toxins and removes tension; if you don't have toxins and tension, you don't need to do the Hatha yoga. It's all curative. But sometimes unconsciously it happens, because of your involvement with things, you might get some toxins and tension. However careful you may be in the kitchen, you may inhale a little smoke if there is a fire there. Sometimes you may, for example, go out to a feast, and since there are people eating, you can't stick to your diet. Often when I go to someone's home, the host wants me to taste something that they have especially prepared, so I have to say yes, at least to satisfy them. And if I eat something like that, and afterward I feel it's a little heavy, I may do a little cleaning. If I am just all by myself, I eat simply; I don't need fancy foods. So in the daily going, you might get some. The mind may be kept always steady, but physically, not always. If you go to the city and stay for a few days, you come back and the lungs feel a little dirty. You may have to do a little more breathing to clean them out. So for the body, it's better to continue the practices, at least in a mild way. The mind, once it is steady, stays there; there's no need to force the mind. But as long as the mind has other desires, you may have a tough time bringing it back again. Once the mind understands everything and knows that that is no good, and this is beautiful, the mind begins to enjoy this. Then, even if you push the mind there, it will say, "Why are you pushing me there? I am happy here. I like to do this." Thus it becomes a habit, and then the mind never gets into trouble.

We have to take time and spend our energy to educate the mind, to make it feel that, "Ah yes, it is much more tasty food than that." No mind will be that foolish to pass up this honey and go for little white sugar. Thankfully, it gets used to this new kind of enjoyment. It may fall back a little due to the old samskaras, so one has to be careful until you are most positive that now no more fences are needed. Like a tree, once it grows stronger, you take away the fence. Otherwise, what is the use of these practices? If you are going to continuously until the death do the same things, then you are gathering firewood, and you don't have time to enjoy the fire. If the mind is educated well, it can take care of everything. It can control the body. Every cell has a consciousness of its own; it can understand. If you are a little weak, the mind will take the upper hand. It's something like a child; if you use the proper tone, he will know that you mean what you say.

Losing yourself.

Amma Claydon, age thirty-eight, married, one of Gurudev's secretaries, ten years practicing yoga.

As far as my daily practice is concerned, I have been practicing meditation in the morning, pranayama, and a few asanas; five or seven, those that suit me the best. I have never failed in my meditation; at least if I have failed, it has been very seldom, but I have been very regular in that. I also consider my work to my guru as one of my practices because I have learned how to do it with a certain attitude, with a certain feeling, which is like part of a spiritual practice. The main thing of how these practices have expressed themselves in my life, what I have learned through them, has been the attitude of service, of which I had not a clue before I started with Swamiji. This attitude of service had never dawned upon me. I had been practicing yoga for many years before I met Swamiji, and it was always sort of a very private thing. That is what has changed my life. I feel that an attitude of service can simplify life to a great degree and make it simple. This attitude makes the understanding wider. It has widened my understanding about life in general, about people, about individuals, and it has made me, most of all, forget myself. That has been the greatest relief in my life, the greatest miracle. I have noticed that I can finally forget myself and that other people and other things are much more important than me. That has made my life very beautiful. I think that I have a very beautiful life because it is full and rewarding, and it has given me a certain degree of peace that has made me able to deal with situations and circumstances that I could have never dealt with in life before. The attitude of service can be expanded to a great number of individuals and can be brought into the family, even married life. It has been that attitude of having been able to forget myself that I think has made me and Arjuna able to relate better to each other than if we were only in a man-woman situation, trying to build a family in a certain way and trying to struggle for the everyday living.

Hearing the guru within.

Swami Atmananda, age twenty-three, head of audio and visual material, Satchidananda Ashram, practicing yoga seven years.

Well, for me, Gurudev's always my example of how a person can live really well. He's an example of how to live, and so I just try to emulate that by having a balanced life and not going to extremes in any activity. I always have Gurudev as a bouncing board; he's my conscience. I've heard him speak so much, in person and on tape and just being around him so much, that he speaks inside me all the time. In everything I do, I hear him. If I think of the whole day, when I'm woken up to meditate and I don't want to go, I ask myself, "Why do I want to meditate?" In that way, the reasons come to me, my mind clears, and I start out on the right side of the bed. And from there, my day begins. I know how I will feel that day if I do meditate or if I don't.

Then I come here for karma yoga, and I try to remember why I'm doing it, what I'm doing it for, and even how I should be doing it. Swamiji always does everything so perfectly. If I don't do it that way, I hear that. I know that I'm kind of copping out, and I know that I'm not putting everything into it. If someone talks to me, I try to listen to what they want, have patience, and understanding. For me, that's the way it is with all of the teachings; I don't think it's anything unique except what helps me the most. It's just that it lasts for a long time, and Gurudev inspires that to last.

Doing what comes up.

Brother Shridar Chaitanya, age twenty-nine, National Co-ordinator Integral Yoga Institutes, yoga practitioner for six years.

The practices mean to me, in terms of my life, that they aren't necessarily formal practices. My formal practices are things which I do as often as possible, and as regularly as possible, but I don't consider them the main emphasis of what I do. To me, the practices are basically moral and ethical teachings by which I try to live. Formal practices may be things which can help me do that better, but without them, I should be able to strive toward a moral and ethical perfection. Certain formal practices such as meditation, pranayama, and asanas help calm my nervous system, make me feel more peaceful, but still, even without those, I feel that I should be able to attain that same feeling, just by how I live life and how I relate to other people. I just do my works as my practice, whatever comes to me, whatever I'm assigned, whatever my responsibilities are. I try to fulfill them in an objective and compassionate way as possible, keeping my peace of mind, and trying not to disturb the peace of mind of others. I never try to let anything disturb me. I just deal with things as they come up, keeping myself flexible so that if something has to be changed, or if some change comes about, I just accept it, and do it if that's necessary.

Ego chopping.

Swami Dharmananda, age twenty-three, runs a natural-food truck for the ashram, yoga practitioner for three years.

Through the practice of yoga I follow in my daily life, it's helped me to live a more happy and more contented life, and it frees me from a lot of attachments that would otherwise be in the mind. I find through doing karma yoga, which is one of the main practices that I do, that it gives me an opportunity to just work for the joy of working, not expecting anything in return; just doing the work for its sake alone. That enables me to keep a more peaceful and a still mind. I also find that having a spiritual master has filled my life very much. Just seeing Gurudev and what he exemplifies has given me a remembrance of something to strive for constantly. That consciousness that he possesses, that being that he is, just keeps me going; that is where I get my strength from, is from his being, and seeing how he is, what a pure instrument he is in God's hands. And I just try to remember that and see what his teachings are, which is to lead basically a dedicated, selfless life and to try to also lead that kind of life to be a pure instrument in his hand. I found that I have a long way to go to do that, but gradually, he slowly is chopping away at this ego, and freeing me, and showing me how to live life as it should be lived.

A calm center.

Sudarshan Anderson, age twenty-nine, married, research assistant in a bacterial-genetics lab.

The practice over seven years now has become so much a part of me that I can hardly make a distinction and say that this is the way that this particular practice is being integrated in my life at this point. I feel as if, through the help of the practices, my whole life has become integrated. It's not so much that the practices are integrated in my life, but that my whole life has become one piece with the help of the practices. They serve to put me in contact with a center around which all of the other aspects of my life can be articulated or co-ordinated. I think that Hatha yoga, meditation, and pranayama, for me, are all very much together. For example, the practice of just sitting in preparation for the meditation is an asana, and it's body consciousness. That awareness that I try to bring to the body is the same kind of awareness that I'm bringing to my body when I'm doing the poses, so that it's a kind of "Hatha awareness." And then there's the breathing, which is very much integrated into the meditation practice also. So the pranayama and the meditation and the body awareness are all the cornerstone of my practice at this point and have been for a long time.

The other practices, for example, the bhakti yoga and the jnana yoga and the karma yoga have always seemed more abstract to me, and in way, I've had more difficulty getting a tangible feel for those, like I have for these other practices. But the breathing, the postures, and the meditation I think have had a profound effect on my workings in the world. As I was saying earlier, I really feel very strongly that they've given me a center around which my whole life has taken a coherent form. Before, there was an awful lot of directions scattered here and there and different impulses, and even at one time, I felt a collection of distinct personalities. Now they seem to have all been integrated around the stable and calm and peaceful awareness that has come about through the meditation and the pranayama. I have also enjoyed, as a matter of course, excellent physical health because of the practices.

A specific example of the integration I was talking about might be just thinking about what I was doing today. I had a whole bunch of sort of routine clean-it-up-and-get-it-together tasks to do at work. I found that while I was doing them I could be perfectly at ease, not at all frustrated or bothered by the fact that I was going to have to spend a half hour doing the same diddly little repetitive task over and over again. I often have to do this on my job, because it's just part of this particular job. Every once in a while you have these stretches of very monotonous little things to do. And I found that I could be perfectly at ease, perfectly relaxed about doing them, without feeling like grumbling, "What with all this training, here I am doing this diddly task." But I can really feel, if I look back, the most striking sense of how the practices have affected my life if I try and compare my life now with the way it was six years ago before the practices were really making any effect. It's just that the overall sense of slow, peace, ease, a kind of happiness that is always there at any minute, and the minute you're not doing something else actively, there's just a sort of sense of well-being that's just there permanently and that's just such a unique sort of joyful feeling that you just can't get over it; it's so great.

Yoga in business.

Hari Zupan, age twenty-eight, single, partner in executive search firm, yoga practitioner for nine years.

The yoga practices including meditation, asanas, on the very physical practice level, make my mind and body much more fit instruments for me to utilize in my work. For example, my energy level is much higher. My ability to deal with people on a calm, even-minded basis is greatly enhanced by the general feeling of peace and calm that I carry with me. Since I'm a kind of salesman, I'm very often subjected to a lot of rejection, repeated factors that would tend to frustrate an indivudual. Thus, there is a constant need for being able to bounce back, to be resilient in the face of failure. And, frankly, if there's one big lesson that yoga has taught me, it is that all failures in life are nothing but stepping stones for your future successes. Especially if you can understand them as such. And I feel that I have understood that to a certain extent so that, for example, when I'm making a sales presentation, if I get a rejection or a failure, as you invariably must, I just move right on to my next presentation, without grumbling, without using that as an excuse to cop-out and quit, and say, "Oh, this business is difficult, or too much." I just keep on going until I'm successful and, in fact, learning to derive the benefit of those failures. In other words, I ask myself why was that particular sales presentation a failure? It was a failure because I failed to do X, Y, or Z. I immediately try to take the responsibility for the failure on myself, rather than trying to blame it on another factor, like the economy is no good, or that person just doesn't know a good thing when they see it. Because what

Swamiji and yoga have taught me is that you must ultimately take responsibility for everything that happens to you, yourself, and that's the only way you can dynamically change your life and the atmosphere around you. It's a constant lesson that's been driven home time after time, because what is the use, after all, of blaming other people and other things? Even if it were somewhat accurate, what difference would it make? You wouldn't be changing anything. You'd merely get the somewhat dubious satisfaction of having pointed the finger elsewhere.

In yoga, I've learned that I, as much as possible, must try to accept the results of my actions as my own responsibility and my own doing and make things better. This has been a very big help in my daily life. I take responsibility for my failures; I learn from the mistakes I've made and apply them to my future actions. This has given me the resiliency to bounce back, even when things get really difficult in the business, and to just keep on going.

Also, another thing I feel I've benefited from in my business, you know, it's not that I can necessarily help everybody that comes to me by finding them a position; some people need to do other things before they can avail themselves of my services. They need to have other experiences; they need to take other approaches, and, frankly, the only time that I get rewarded financially for any of my counseling is upon actual placement of an individual. So I see many people take the attitude in my business, if you understand in the first two minutes that you can't place them, give them a polite kiss-off and good-bye, and don't spend anymore time with them. But I have understood them, from being in that position of looking for a job, how difficult it is, and what a sensitive position you are in, and how a little bit of kindness and good constructive advice, even if it isn't the final advice that will land one the job, it can be very important and very much of a boost on that path of finding a job. So I always endeavor to offer whatever concrete advice, frank and honest suggestions as I can to an individual, even understanding that although my business is very much profit-oriented and results-oriented, in terms of placement and commission, that I'm also

292

there to perform a service. If somebody comes into my office, I'm performing a service, and I can take it as such. I have the opportunity to help an individual, even though it's not going to be a directly remunerative act, which is something else I've learned from the art of karma yoga; where you learn to do things not just for the results that you can measure in terms of dollars and cents, or any other way. In other words, forgetting yourself for the moment, your own personal need, desire, and want, and just helping and serving whomever comes before you; which I have been able to apply in my business to a certain extent, and that's also been very helpful and wonderful. Doing karma yoga is serving, not thinking of yourself; but a funny thing happens, even though you are not thinking of yourself, you get a certain reward from being selfless, which you don't even expect, unless you remember from time to time what the joy is of actually doing something, just for the pure sake of serving. And that joy is one I am able to experience very often in my work, thanks to yoga.

A clean closet.

Brahman Berman, age twenty-six, married, diesel mechanic, practicing yoga five years.

The main thing which I see I am working toward is perfection in action. That's the way I see the practices. Being mechanically oriented, I relate to most things on a mechanical basis. For example, the body. It's like a finely tuned machine, and so the way I want my body to function is the same way you would want an automobile to function. The way I integrate the practices into my life is by trying not to do anything which might interfere with the functioning of my personal vehicle, my body. That means screening out certain things, basic things which intoxicate and pollute the body, like smoking, drinking, etc. Then also there is, of course, mental disturbance. There are circumstances that cause the mind to become toxic and polluted: things like extremely violent situations, violent movements, and pornographic movies, which might cause a lot of disturbance. But in the broader scheme, I'm interested in just how I'm affecting my family and everything around me. Right now I'm trying to become as stable and as efficient as possible. I would like to feel as I walk down the path that I'm not leaving a mess behind me, that there's no clutter that I'm going to have to go back and correct. Because the way I'm treading the path right now, *this is it;* this is the only chance I've got. I'm not going to be given the opportunities to correct my mistakes later on. I probably will make lots of mistakes, but if I have the attitude of perfection in front of me, then I know that what I'm doing now is right, and I won't have to worry about whether I'll get that desire tomorrow or next year. It's sort of trying to deal with all the present situations and handle them in the right attitude. It's a refinement right now, trying to make sure that everything is fit and functioning well. So, if I deal with it in that respect, whether it comes to washing the dishes, or cleaning the house, I try to deal with it as soon as possible. The practices and the teachings are designed to make me more fit to deal with these things right now, and not let them build up. That to me seems the way I have to live my life. It makes it a very simple existence. It seems that the simplicity of the life-style makes for a happier attitude. If I get really involved with a lot of disturbing things and start falling behind, it becomes a lot of clutter. It's like a closet which you never want to go into because it's such a mess. That's pretty much how I see it.

Letting go.

Shakti Berman, age twenty-three, married, mother, yoga practitioner for four years.

I think on a day-to-day level, the thing that has taken over my life the most is just remembering that there's a reason and a purpose to work on oneself. In terms of Hatha yoga and meditation, that's really on an irregular basis, maybe once a week, if I can get to that. I do it on days that I'm really full of stress and tension but, most of the time, just maintaining house and keeping up with the child is a lot. The biggest obstacle I have is in surrendering to things which happen to come into my life, causing me to be impatient in those situations. The teachings have given me the ability to cope better, to feel dispassion where there once was a lot of attachment. On a specific level, I've been able to apply the practices to being a mother. Doing it has been hard, especially being a mother, being on demand all of the time. Sometimes there's a trigger inside that says, "I just can't tolerate this; I just can't give it a single minute more." But I feel that I'm learning, that I'm continuing to go in, and becoming non-attached to whatever it was I wanted to be doing. Because of that, there's a result, an element of peace that comes in, letting go all of the time. And each single time that I do it, it works; and because it works, I keep doing it more and more. The times that I don't give in, that I can't let go, it's because I'm not allowing that inner voice to say loud enough what it is that will bring me peace. I'm blocking it out, saying, "No, I won't listen to you. This time I'm not going to listen." But that's what's nice; you hear it louder and louder and louder, and you hear it more and more and more. Before, you had to look for it, but now it's a lot easier to just be quiet and listen. There were so many opinions going on inside of me that I was torn at every situation. I had some kind of opinion about every person that I dealt with; how they should be, or how they shouldn't be. Today, this week, this month, that's the thing from which I'm feeling the greatest relief. I don't have to be so involved with all that. There's more of a security in being with my ownself.

Another thing that's happening lately is in the way that I look at myself. It's like a mirror that has been turned toward me so that I see those past attitudes falling away. Thank goodness I didn't see it before they started to fall away, because I probably would have been aghast at the vanity involved in the way I relate to people, and the way I think people relate to me. There was, and still is, a lot of involvement with my physical appearance. But now I see two or three more aspects of those attitudes, and by seeing them, it's easier to just say, "Oh, boy!" It's good to see them because now they're not quite as much a part of me, and I'm able to look at them a little further off. And that's a big relief too. It really makes me feel the Guru. I'm not always in tune with what the Guru is, but lately I've been feeling a force outside of myself that's aiding my evolution, and I keep hearing the phrase that says if you take one step toward the Guru, the Guru takes ten toward you. I really feel that.

A mother's love.

Radha Sackett, age twenty-five, married, mother, yoga practitioner for six years.

As far as bhakti yoga goes, being a mother has just about put the icing on the cake. For me, a mother's love is the purest kind of love; it's almost purer than love of God. I've heard that it's next to love of God, not quite as high. I remember before, when I loved God intensely, but now, I've almost forgotten about God, and all my love is going out to this child. I'm with her all the time, and it just happens to be where my love goes. It's just purified much more, and it hasn't brought the least amount of pain, so I know that it must be some kind of detached pure loving, even though it feels so attached. It's really a lesson in bhakti yoga, really putting it into practice, because I have this deity right here in front of me all the time. When you love something really intensely, like your child, it gives you the energy and the awareness to purify all your motives and actions. You don't want to hurt this thing, not in the slightest or subtlest way. Often, you may see yourself hurt it in tiny ways, and so you try to purify those things as they come along. Being a wife of course involves more obstacles, because a grown adult isn't as pure as an infant, and so your love may have more obstacles along the way. Your husband or wife should be someone who you really see God in a lot, and from whom you get energy to purify yourself. How not to get disturbed about things is what yoga is really about, and there's just so many opportunities in a householding life to learn that, it's just an everyday bust. It's hard to even think of it as yoga anymore. You learn a lot that way.

Japa yoga and other practices have really gone by the way-side, at least temporarily. I'm sure the practices would help, like after nine months or so, but when your baby's first born, for this time, you're really sailing, and you don't need much in the way of practices like a mantra. After that, though, you start to need it more, and then it's really difficult to get back into it; but it's only necessary when you really feel that you are being disturbed in your daily activities, and the mind starts to wander crazily.

A friend's love.

Subadra Clark, single, age thirty-eight, guidance counselor, four years experience in yoga.

When I decided to practice brahmacharya, it helped me grow to like men as friends, and it really cut out a lot of exploitation that I was into. I didn't know any other way to be with men. That's been a big change this year, to really learn to like men as people. I couldn't relate to them. I had lots of women friends, and I had lots of men friends, but I wasn't truly friends with them. So that's been a relief, and it's been a specific help. I hear myself saying things now truly compassionate about men; and for all these years I've been fighting men—"Oh, damn men, they've got it so good; women have been taking the brunt for such a long time"—and now I can really appreciate how men are caught in life, in so much stuff. Maybe more than women, especially the men of my generation don't have the options of exploring as many things as I've had the chance to. They're locked in their careers, in fulfilling their parents' expectations for them to be successful people; they're locked into earning the income for the family.

The integration within.

Arjuna Claydon, age twenty-eight, married, general handyman and student, practicing yoga four years.

Since the beginning, I've always tried to make the yoga practices the focal point of each day. For me though, there are certain parts of the day that are more formally given to the practices like meditation, pranayama, and Hatha yoga. I have to set some time aside for them because you just can't grab them on the run, as you would a cheese sandwich at the office. So there's sort of a feeling in my life of having to give a certain amount of time for whatever it is that I'm doing, or whatever process I'm going through with my wife and our situation. I try to give the practices my utmost attention so that I feel the effects and the results that come out of doing them. I not only try to keep a separate part of the day for formal practices, but also to hang in there and not get worried. I guess that's important, and I see it's important because I see the results in whatever it is that I'm doing. I know for instance that if I back off from the yoga practices, that after a while, I'll notice that my habits change a little bit. But with the practices, those same actions are done in a slightly different, cooled-out, together, more observant sort of fashion. That ranges over every type of activity that I engage in, so that by seeing the results, you are encouraged to stay with it. You know the benefits intimately in your relationships with people, the kind of work you do, the quality you turn out; yoga has something to do with that. Everything, even driving the car, it all becomes obvious what benefits you've attained to. And then also, there are a lot of times when you are just doing something, any daily activity, no matter what it is, when you might feel that you're ready to take on more in a formal sense, and you get into a philosophical place that you have at your quiet moments, and you think over and compare your life as it is, and as it has been, and as it might be; and you sort of make some constant value adjustments about the value of the practices in your life.

So I'd say after four years of relatively constant practice and thinking things over, I can see from week to week how my head changes. The more often the changes occur, the less I feel I can say about it, because the more that's happening is not available for words. It's a very subjective experience, but that's the real integration, how the thought processes and the attitudes form your ideas; how you use your life; how you act in life; how you integrate your practices into your everyday activities; and how daily activities become the practices in their own way. It's like saying, "I have to do more Hatha yoga." It becomes obvious when you have to do more Hatha yoga. When I have to meditate more, I guess to some people it isn't obvious, but to me it is obvious, constantly. The more meditation I do, the better off I'll be, because that's what needs to be fed, that's the real nitty gritty on which everything rests.

Beyond the ego clashes.

Shanti, age twenty-seven, single, one of Gurudev's secretaries, practicing yoga for eight years.

At this point, I would honestly say that my mental attitude is that whatever is given to me to do, I try to do it the best I can. I've gone through the mental attitude of trying to do it great, for the sake of doing it great, and getting off on that. That game has kind of slid away, even though I still get off on it sometimes. Really, who cares already? Whatever is given to you to do, just try to do it as well as possible, and think of all the things that are involved in it. Just do it and try to enjoy it, and if it has to do with someone else, make it as beautiful and sweet as possible. I've gone beyond the point of even consciously trying to avoid ego clashes. You go through a time where you are so concerned that if you do an action a certain way, then your ego will be involved. We all have egos, so just try and accept it. If I have an ego, so what? At least let people see my ego. They have one, and I have one; we're just trying to make them nice. After a while, you just drop the attitude that you don't have an ego, and you just try to slowly whittle it away. Saying, okay, I'm going to let go of my ego; I'm going to stop trying to beat it away; I'll just be here and do what I'm given. Somehow, if you put yourself in your guru's hands or in divine hands, you really feel that. Then you can just let go of all your conscious wondering of where you're at.

Glossary of Common Sanskrit Terms

Adharma
Contrary to the law and to what is right; demerit.

Advaita
Non-dualism.

Aham
I; the ego.

Aham Kara
Egoism or self-conceit; self-consciousness of "I."

Ahimsa
Non-injury in thought, word, and deed.

Ajapa japa
The mantra goes on by itself without any conscious effort.

Ajna-cakra
Sixth chakra, opposite the eyebrows, the seat of the mind.

Akasa
Ether.

Akhanda

Unbroken, i.e., Akhanda japa—japa said for a long period of time.

Anahata

The fourth chakra opposite the heart; also mystic inner sound.

Ananda

Bliss; joy.

Annam

Food and matter.

Apana

The nerve current which originates from the anus and governs the abdomen. It is a downward-flowing energy.

Arati

A ritual service done to God with camphor lamps and ringing of bells.

Asana

Posture or seat.

Ashrama

Monastery; also order of life (i.e., the four ashramas, brahmacharya or studentship, grhastha or householder life, vanaprasta or retiring, and sanyasa or monastic life.)

Ashtanga Yoga

Raja yoga's eight-limbed path.

Asteya

One of the five parts of the yamas, non-stealing.

Atma

The Self.

Bandha

Certain advanced Hatha yoga techniques, done in conjunction with some pranayamas.

Basti
> The yogic enema, done by sucking water up through the bowels.

Bhagavan
> The Lord.

Bhakta
> Devotee.

Bhakti
> Devotion, love of God.

Bhava or Bhavana
> Used to describe different spiritual attitudes, i.e., Santa bhava—peaceful attitude.

Bija
> Seed or source.

Bindu
> The point of origin from which everything has manifested.

Brahma
> God as creator (See Vishnu and Siva).

Brahmachari
> The first ashrama: the celibate student.

Brahman
> I quote from Sivananda: "The Absolute Reality; the Truth proclaimed in the Upanishads; the Supreme eternal; all-pervading, changeless, Existence; Existence-knowledge-bliss-absolute; the substratum of Jiva, Ishwara, and Maya; Absolute Consciousness; it is not only all-powerful, but all power itself; not only all-knowing and blissful, but all knowledge and bliss itself."

Buddha
> The enlightened one.

Buddhi
> Intellect; understanding.

Chakra
Plexus or subtle nerve center.

Chitta
Mind-stuff, what the mind is made of.

Dasa
Slave or servant.

Daya
Compassion.

Dharma
Righteous way, virtue.

Dhyana
Meditation.

Diksha
Initiation.

Gita
Song; refers to the sacred scripture, the Bhagavad Gita.

Grhastha
Householder.

Guna
Quality born of nature.

Guru
Teacher; master.

Hari
A deity that destroys evil deeds; another name for Krishna.

Hatha yoga
Yoga for gaining control over the body.

Ida
Nerve current which terminates at the left nostril; cooling nerve fiber. (See Pingala.)

Ishta Devata
> Favorite deity.

Jagat guru
> World teacher.

Japa
> Repetition of God's name.

Jaya
> Victory, mastery.

Jiva
> Individual soul with ego.

Jivan mukta
> One liberated while living.

Jnana
> Knowledge or wisdom of the absolute.

Jnana yoga
> Path of knowledge; thinking seriously on the true nature of the Self.

Jyotih
> An effulgent light.

Karma
> Action. Three kinds; sanchita—all accumulated actions; parabdha—that portion of karma that must be worked out in a particular lifetime; and kriyaman—current karma being performed.

Karma yoga
> The yoga of selfless action; service to humanity.

Kriya
> Physical action; also particular cleansing procedures in Hatha yoga.

Kriya yoga
Yoga of action; yoga of self-purification through external service or worship. Also a special path followed by followers of Paramahamsa Yogananda.

Kundalini
The elemental cosmic energy within the individual; like a serpent it rests coiled at the base of the spine.

Layayoga
The process of absorption of the individual soul into the supreme soul; another name for nada yoga and kundalini yoga.

Lila
Play; sport; the cosmos looked upon as a divine play.

Maharsi
Great sage.

Mahatma
Great soul; saint; sage.

Mala
Rosary used for counting numbers of japa.

Mandala
Region; sphere or plane.

Manipura chakra
The third chakra centered around the region of the navel.

Mantra
Sacred syllable or word or set of words designed for contemplation through mental repetition.

Marga
Path; road.

Mauna
Silence.

Maya
> The illusive power of Brahman; the veiling and projective power of the universe.

Moksha
> Release; liberation from the bondage of karma and the wheel of death and rebirth.

Mudra
> Symbols shown by hands during worship; also a certain type of Hatha yoga.

Muladhara
> The lowermost of the six yogic centers in the body.

Muni
> A sage.

Nada
> The mystic and primal sound; the first vibration from which all has manifested.

Nadi
> Subtle nerve fiber for the psychic current.

Narayana
> A proper name of God; it means one who pervades all things.

Nauli
> Hatha yoga kriya, where the abdomen is churned by the rotation of the recti muscles.

Neti
> Hatha yoga kriya for cleansing the nose, by passing a string through the nostrils and out the mouth.

Neti-Neti
> Means "Not this; not this," an analytical process by which all names and forms are progressively negated to arrive at the eternal underlying truth.

Nirvana
Liberation.

Niyama
The second step in the raja yoga eightfold path.

Ojas
Vigor—spiritual energy, vitality—developed through the creative power of celibacy and spiritual practice.

Om
The sacred syllable symbolizing Brahma; sound of the universe.

Padmasana
The lotus pose, a meditative posture.

Para
Supreme.

Parabhakti
Supreme devotion to God, where the devotee sees his deity everywhere. Here devotion transcends all form and rituals.

Pingala
A nadi which terminates at the right nostril, heating nerve fiber. (See Ida)

Prana
Vital energy.

Pratyahara
Withdrawal of the senses from their objects; fifth limb of the eight-limbed path.

Prema
Divine love (for God).

Puja
Worship.

Purusa
Self which abides in the heart of all things.

Rajas
One of the three gunas. The principle of dynamism in nature bringing about all change; this quality generates with an individual passion and restlessness.

Raja yoga
The science of mental control and meditation; propounded by Patanjali; ashtanga yoga.

Sadhana
Self-effort; spiritual practice.

Sadhu
Pious or righteous man.

Sakti
Absolute power, cosmic energy. Another name for the divine mother.

Samadhi
Oneness, the mind becomes identified with the object of meditation; superconscious state where absolute is experienced with complete understanding and joy.

Samsara
Life through repeated death and rebirth.

Samskara
Impression within the mind; prenatal tendency.

Samyama
Perfect restraint; complete condition of balance and repose; last three rungs on eight-limbed path: concentration, meditation, and samadhi.

Santa or Shanthi
Peaceful; calm.

Sanyasa
Renunciation of worldy life; last of the ashramas.

Satchidananda
Existence-knowledge-bliss-absolute.

Satsanga
Association with the wise (good).

Satvaguna
Quality of light, purity, and goodness.

Satya
Truth; Brahman or the Absolute.

Siddhi
Psychic power.

Soucha
Purity (internally and externally); cleanliness.

Sushumna
The nerve current that passes through the spinal column through which the kundalini rises.

Sutra
An aphorism with minimum words and maximum sense; a terse sentence.

Swadharma
One's prescribed duty in life according to the eternal law.

Swadhaya
Study of the religious scriptures.

Tamas
Ignorance; inertia; darkness.

Tantra
A particular spiritual path laying great emphasis on japa and puja.

Tapas
Austerity and purificatory action; also acceptance of pain without return.

Vairagya
Indifference; dispassion toward worldly enjoyments.

Veda
The most ancient and authentic scripture of the Hindus.

Vedanta
School of Hindu thought based on the Vedas that expresses non-dualism in its conditional and unconditional aspects. Literally means, the end of the Vedas; the Upanishads.

Viveka
Discrimination between real and unreal; between Self and non-Self.

Vritti
Thought wave; mental modification.

Yama
The first limb of raja yoga; restraint.

Yoga
Union with the Supreme Being; also the process of union of the practitioner with the universal soul.

Yogi
One who practices yoga, who strives earnestly for union with God.

NOTE: Some of these terms (along with many more) can be found in Swami Sivananda's Yoga-Vedanta Dictionary.

o